# Syllabus of Gynecologic Pathology with Clinical Correlations

# SYLLABUS OF GYNECOLOGIC PATHOLOGY WITH CLINICAL CORRELATIONS

**Tung Van Dinh, M.D., FACOG, FASCP**
Professor of Gynecology-Obstetrics and Pathology
Department of Obstetrics and Gynecology
The University of Texas Medical Branch
Galveston, Texas

Foreword by
**J. Donald Woodruff, M.D., FACOG**
Emeritus Professor of Gynecology and Gynecologic Pathology
Johns Hopkins School of Medicine
Baltimore, Maryland

**University of Texas Press Austin**

Printed in the United States of America

First edition, 1990



♾ The paper used in this publication meets the minimum requirements of American National Standard for Information Sciences—Permanence of Paper for Printed Library Materials, ANSI Z39.48-1984.

**Library of Congress Cataloging-in-Publication Data**

Dinh, Tung Van, 1930–
Syllabus of gynecologic pathology with clinical correlations / Tung Van Dinh ; foreword by J. Donald Woodruff. — 1st ed.
p. cm.
Includes bibliographical references.
ISBN 0-292-77632-2 (alk. paper)
1. Generative organs, Female—Diseases—Outlines, syllabi, etc. I. Title.
[DNLM: 1. Genital Diseases, Female—pathology—outlines. WP 18 D584s]
RG112.D56 1990
618.1′07—dc20
DNLM/DLC
for Library of Congress 89-70559
CIP

**To my wife, Tonia To,**
**and my children,**
**Tuan, Tue, Tri, and Tho,**
**for their constant love,**
**support, and understanding**

# Contents


Foreword ix
Preface xi
1. The Vulva 1
2. The Urethra 26
3. The Vagina 30
4. The Cervix 40
5. The Endometrium 56
6. The Myometrium 71
7. The Fallopian Tubes 81
8. The Ovary: Inflammations, Non-neoplastic Lesions, Abnormal Gonadal Sex Differentiation, and Premature Ovarian Failure 92
9. Generalities on Ovarian Neoplasms 104
10. Epithelial Tumors of the Ovary 109
11. Germ Cell Tumors of the Ovary 121
12. Gonadal Stromal Tumors of the Ovary 132
13. Miscellaneous Tumors of the Ovary 139
14. Diseases of the Mesosalpinx and Uterine Ligaments 145
15. The Placenta 147
Index 165

# Figures

1. Different concepts of microinvasive carcinoma of the vulva 19
2. Different concepts of microinvasive carcinoma of the cervix 47

# Foreword

Clinical correlation with the gross and microscopic pathology is important in every branch of medicine; however, it is particularly significant in the female genital canal. The misinterpretations of HPV infection of the lower genital canal, the problem with differentiation of endometrial hyperplasia and cancer, and the confusion surrounding ovarian neoplasia are only a few of the complicated features of pathology in the female generative tract. Consequently, it is of major importance that such a syllabus as prepared by Tung Van Dinh be introduced into our society.

Dr. Dinh has been interested in gyn pathology since he first visited the Johns Hopkins School of Medicine in 1960–1961. He, at that time, spent a year in the gyn pathology laboratory, and his enthusiasm for this subspecialty was demonstrated by his efforts to introduce biweekly reviews of specialized topics into the regular program. Although he returned to DaNang to carry on his work for his people, his enthusiasm for gyn pathology apparently never waned. His return to the United States at the end of the Vietnam War was made possible through the dedicated support of certain friends at the University of Texas Medical Branch in Galveston. Tung accepted this challenge with vigor, and his expertise is demonstrated by the fact that in a decade he has been promoted from a staff member to professor in the Departments of Obstetrics-Gynecology and Pathology. His syllabus is just another demonstration of his enthusiasm and dedication. The volume is carefully prepared, and the theses are well documented. It is concise and should become a prominent volume in the library of every gynecologist and gynecologic pathologist, since both must be indoctrinated in the intricacies of relationships.

Dr. Dinh is to be congratulated on the development of the easily read and very complete thesis.

J. Donald Woodruff, M.D.
Johns Hopkins Hospital
Baltimore, Maryland

# Preface

The concept of this syllabus came from my residents, who wanted a core textbook that contained the essentials of gynecologic pathology to be used for review after lectures and before exams. I chose the outline format for its conciseness; the illustrations it lacks can be found elsewhere, in the many excellent textbooks and atlases available. This syllabus has been used successfully in our residency program for the past seven years. It represents the core of knowledge in gynecologic pathology that a gynecologist must master for good practice of the specialty.

I owe a special debt of gratitude to Dr. J. D. Woodruff of the Johns Hopkins School of Medicine, whose teaching, in 1960, inspired in me a love of the science of gynecologic pathology and who has continued to teach me since, and to Dr. William McGanity, former chairman of the Department of Obstetrics and Gynecology at the University of Texas Medical Branch, who supported and directed my retraining in obstetrics, gynecology, and pathology after my arrival in this country in 1975.

I would also like to express my thanks to the editorial staff of the University of Texas Press, who choose to remain anonymous and who have provided invaluable assistance and superb collaboration in the production of this book. Finally, special thanks are due to Mrs. Lynne Matous, who labored through repeated typings of my manuscript.

Tung Van Dinh, M.D.

# Syllabus of Gynecological Pathology with Clinical Correlations

# 1. The Vulva

I. Embryology
II. Histology
III. Frequent dermatoses
IV. Vulvar lesions in systemic diseases
V. Infections
VI. Benign tumors
VII. Non-neoplastic epithelial disorders
VIII. Neoplastic intraepithelial disorders
IX. Invasive malignancies

## I. Embryology

- External genitalia begin with an undifferentiated stage at 4 weeks: genital tubercle, urogenital folds, labioscrotal swellings. All are of ectodermal origin.
- Sexual characteristics begin at 9 weeks; external genital organs are fully formed at 12 weeks.
- Genital tubercle becomes clitoris; urogenital folds become labia minora; labioscrotal swellings become labia majora, mons pubis, and posterior commissure.
- Bartholin's glands: outgrowths of the urogenital sinus (endoderm), equivalent to bulbourethral glands in males.
- Vestibule: region between hymeneal ring and labia minora, bounded by the fourchette posteriorly; the vagina and urethra open into it; endodermal in origin.

## II. Histology (*skin*)

### A. Labia majora

1. ***Epidermis* lined by stratified squamous epithelium.**
2. ***Dermis* with hair follicles and three types of glands:**
   a. *Merocrine or eccrine glands* (sweat glands).
   b. *Holocrine glands* (sebaceous glands).
   c. *Apocrine glands* with "decapitation secretion" specific to vulva, perianal area, axilla, and breast; begin to secrete cyclically at menarche. Composed of large cells with pink staining cytoplasm.

### B. Labia minora:

differ from labia majora by the absence of the granular layer of the epithelium, the absence of hair follicles, the paucity of apocrine glands, and the presence of sebaceous glands opening directly onto the surface of skin.

### C. Clitoris

- Consists of two corpora cavernosa.
- Differs from the penis by the absence of corpus spongiosum.

### D. Bartholin's glands *(major vestibular glands)*

- Acini: mucus-secreting columnar epithelium.
- Duct: transitional epithelium.
- Orifice of duct: stratified epithelium (similar to that of vagina).
- Minor vestibular glands: around vestibule.
- Only area of the female genital canal of endodermal origin.

### E. Urethra

- Lined by transitional epithelium with stratified epithelium at the orifice.
- Skene's ducts (not glands) at orifice of urethra, lined by squamous epithelium.

## III. Frequent dermatoses

### A. Contact dermatitis

- Due to local irritants: perfumes, sprays, synthetic fibers, vaginal contraceptives, etc.
- Red, edematous, inflamed skin.
- Treatment: eliminate offending factors; topical cortisone preparations for itching.

### B. Chronic dermatitis

- Gross: whitish, grayish, or reddish lesion (similar to old hyperplastic dystrophy).
- Microscopic: hyperkeratosis, acanthosis, chronic inflammatory infiltrate.
- Treatment: fluorinated corticosteroids as lotions or creams, subcutaneous injection of triamcinolone (Woodruff).

### C. Intertrigo

- Fissure of macerated skin in the intercrural and interlabial folds in obese patients.
- Treatment: avoid moisture, relieve obesity.

### D. Psoriasis

- Gross: erythematous plaques covered by fine silvery scales (Auspitz's sign). Plaques can be present in other areas of the body. In vulva, lesions can be masked by moisture and resemble a nonspecific dermatitis.

- Microscopic: parakeratosis, rete pegs elongated and clubbed, thin suprapapillary plates, capillary prominent in dermal papillae, Munro abscesses in epidermis.
- Treatment: fluorinated corticosteroids.

### E. Tinea cruris

- Superficial infection of groin and upper thighs by dermatophytic fungi, often associated with tinea elsewhere (toes, etc.).
- Itching, red lesion.
- Treatment: imidazoles.

### F. Lichen planus

- Gross: flat violaceous papules, often white plaques on vulva, may involve vagina.
- Microscopic: hyperkeratosis, acanthosis, bandlike infiltrate of lymphocytes hugging the epidermis.
- Treatment: corticosteroid creams.

## IV. Vulvar lesions in systemic diseases

### A. Crohn's disease

- Rarely affects the vulva.
- Gross: formation of rectoperineal or rectovaginal fistulas and draining sinuses.
- Microscopic: inflammatory infiltrate and non-caseating granulomas.
- Treatment: therapy for Crohn's disease (antibiotics, metronidazole, and steroids) before and after repair of fistulas.

### B. Behcet's disease

- Cause: still unknown; autoimmune or viral.
- Characterized by a triple symptom complex: ulcerations in mouth, external genitalia, and eye.

- Histology: intense inflammatory infiltrate and vasculitis with occlusion of many vessels.
- Treatment: corticosteroids.

**C. Diabetes mellitus:** vulvitis often due to monilial infection.

**D. Chronic anemia:** vulvar ulceration.

**E. Uremia:** brownish yellow patches on the external genitals (uremic frost).

### F. Tuberculosis of vulva

- Rare, caused by Mycobacterium tuberculosis.
- Due to direct inoculation from an infected sexual partner, or to autoinoculation by hematogenous or direct spread (fallopian tube, endometrium).
- Gross: ulcerated nodule at labia or in vestibular region with irregular and ragged borders.
- Microscopic: classic caseating tubercles with acid-fast bacilli.
- Treatment: antituberculosis drugs.

## V. Infections

### A. Syphilis

- Venereal disease caused by Treponema pallidum, anaerobic spirochete.
- Diagnosis by darkfield microscopy, serologic tests (RPR, VDRL), and FTA-ABS (fluorescent labeled treponema antibody absorption).
- Treatment: benzathine penicillin or tetracycline; benzathine penicillin or erythromycin during pregnancy.

#### 1. Primary lesion *(chancre)*

- Incubation 3 weeks.
- Gross: painless firm lesion with an ulcer-

ated center; can be multiple, located on the labia or at the introitus, non-tender inguinal lymphadenitis.

- Microscopic: acute and chronic inflammation, marked perivascular inflammatory response, large number of plasma cells, spirochete demonstrable in lesion.

2. **Secondary lesion *(condyloma lata)***
   - Appears 6 weeks to 6 months after primary lesion.
   - Gross: plateau-like excrescence, grayish necrotic appearance.
   - Microscopic: acanthosis, epithelial hyperplasia, chronic inflammatory cells with many plasma cells, arteritis, spirochete demonstrable in lesion.

3. **Tertiary lesion *(gumma or ulcer)***
   - Rare.
   - Appears several months or years after inoculation.
   - Microscopic: granuloma with giant cells, epithelioid and mononuclear cells; prominent endothelial proliferation and thickening of vascular walls. Plasma cell infiltration conspicuous.

### B. Chancroid

- Rare, caused by Hemophilus ducreyi, a gram-negative, nonmotile bacillus demonstrated in smears and cultures.
- Incubation: 3–10 days.
- Gross: solitary or multiple ulcerations ragged and irregular with inguinal adenitis; soft chancre is painful and tender.
- Microscopic: chronic inflammation with lymphocytes and plasma cells.

- Diagnosis by gram stain and culture of purulent material.
- Treatment: erythromycin or trimethoprim-sulfamethoxazole.

## C. Granuloma inguinale *(donovanosis)*

- Rare, caused by Calymmatobacterium granulomatis, a gram-negative encapsulated rod of Enterobacteriaceae family.
- Incubation: 1–12 weeks.
- Gross: begins as a small tender papule and spreads by superficial ulceration along the inguinal pubic areas as painless ulcers with rolled borders. Possible premalignant lesion in chronic state (necessity of biopsy).
- Microscopic: chronic inflammation with histiocytes (granuloma cells), sometimes pseudo-epitheliomatous hyperplasia with bizarre acanthosis, abnormal maturation at rete tips; Donovan bodies in large vacuolated histiocytes.
- Diagnosis: Donovan bodies in large mononuclear cells (resemble closed safety pins in Wright's or Giemsa stains) found in smears or specimens taken from ulcers.
- Treatment: tetracycline, ampicillin, chloramphenicol prescribed for 2–3 weeks.

## D. Lymphogranuloma venereum *(Lymphopathia venereum)*

- Caused by Chlamydia trachomatis type L.
- Incubation: 4–21 days.
- Gross: begins with an often-overlooked small ulcerated lesion and pronounced inguinal adenitis; progressing to vulvar edema and draining sinuses leading to rectal and urethral strictures. Malignant potential in chronic state (necessity of biopsy).

- Microscopic: infiltration with large mononuclear and plasma cells, dilatation of lymphatic vessels and endothelial proliferation; pseudo-epitheliomatous hyperplasia can be seen.
- Diagnosis by complement fixation test and culture of pus.
- Treatment: tetracycline, doxycycline, erythromycin, for 3–6 weeks; aspiration of fluctuant lymph nodes (no incision and drainage).

## E. Herpes

- Common infection due to herpes simplex virus, variety Hominis type II or I.
- Incubation: 3–7 days.
- Gross: vesicles, then very painful ulcers, associated sometimes with edema of vulva and enlarged, tender inguinal nodes.
- Biopsy: eosinophilic intranuclear inclusions.
- Cytology: cells with ground glass multinuclei (primary), intranuclear inclusions (secondary).
- Diagnosis mostly by cytology and cultures.
- Treatment: Betadine locally, acyclovir systemically.
- Cesarean section should be performed in pregnant women if there are active lesions or a positive culture within 2 weeks of predicted delivery.

## F. Molluscum contagiosum

- Due to a pox virus.
- Gross: tumors 5–8 mm with umbilicated center, pruriginous, mostly in clusters.
- Microscopic: acanthosis, invagination of the epidermis (central dimple) with cells containing inclusion bodies (molluscum bodies).
- Treatment: curettage or electrocauterization.
- Lesions can regress spontaneously.

## G. Condylomata acuminata

- Common lesion caused by human papilloma virus (often HPV 6/11).
- Incubation: 1–8 months, average 3 months.
- Gross: solitary or multiple pointed excrescences over vulva.
- Microscopic: hyperkeratosis, parakeratosis, papillomatosis, acanthosis, perinuclear halo, and chronic dermal inflammation.
- Treatment: topical podophylline or trichloracetic acid, laser surgery, electrocauterization, cryocauterization.
- Cesarean section should be performed in multiple condylomata acuminata (lacerations). Laryngeal papilloma in newborn not prevented by cesarean section.
- Do not perform biopsy of condylomata acuminata after podophyllin treatment because the lesion can mimic carcinoma in situ. (After treatment wait at least 2 weeks before biopsy.)

## H. Hidradenitis suppurativa

- Infection of apocrine glands by Staphylococcus aureus.
- Deep-seated painful subcutaneous nodules which can become confluent draining masses, similar lesions in axillae.
- Treatment: unroofing incisions or wide excision of the infected skin and antibiotics.

## I. Fox Fordyce disease

- Due to apocrine gland obstruction.
- Gross: tiny, elevated, firm pruritic papules.
- Microscopic: inflammatory infiltrate, dilatation of acini, exudation of secretion into adjacent tissue.

- Treatment: oral contraceptives and local anti-pruritic medications.

### J. Vestibular adenitis

- Minor vestibular glands extend as a ring around the introitus.
- Inflammation causes burning pain and dyspareunia.
- Transitional epithelium of ducts can be mistaken for carcinoma in situ in biopsies.
- Treatment: excision if symptomatic.

## VI. Benign tumors

### A. Cystic

#### 1. Bartholin's duct cyst

- Due to obstruction and dilatation of duct.
- Cyst is lined by transitional epithelium or flattened epithelium from the vicinity of the mucus-secreting acini of Bartholin's gland.
- Treatment: marsupialization or use of Word catheter maintained for 4–6 weeks.
- Can be infected with Neisseria, Staphylococcus, or other agents and become Bartholin's abscess.

#### 2. Mucus cysts *(dysontogenetic cysts)*

- Lined by a cuboidal or columnar mucous-secreting epithelium.
- Arise from remnants of the urogenital sinus or vestibular glands.
- Treatment: excision.

#### 3. Cysts of the canal of Nuck in inguinal canal *(peritoneum-lined cysts or hydrocele in vulva)*

- Analogous to the hydrocele of the spermatic cord.

- Found in labium majus or in inguinal canal.
- Arise from inclusions of the peritoneum along the round ligament.
- Treatment: excision (diagnostic differential to exclude hernia, enlarged inguinal nodes, ectopic testes).

4. **Epidermal inclusion cysts**
   - Lined by a smooth layer of keratinizing squamous epithelium; cyst contains thick, cheesy material.
   - Due to obstruction of the sebaceous gland duct or traumatic inclusion of the epithelium (episiotomy).
   - Treatment: excision if symptomatic.

## B. Solid

1. **Acrochordon *(skin tag, fibroepithelial polyp)***
   - Gross: benign tumor, pedunculated or not, can reach large size.
   - Microscopic: normal epidermis with loose fibrous connective tissue stroma (fat and vessels).
   - Treatment: excision if symptomatic or if there is concern about malignancy.
2. **Hemangioma**
   - Gross: reddish, tiny lesions (cherry angiomata).
   - Microscopic: numerous dilated capillaries lined by a single layer of endothelial cells.
   - No treatment required, unless bleeding (surgery, cryocautery, or laser).
3. **Fibroma and lipofibroma**
   - Gross: lesion firm and smooth with a whitish or grayish color.

- Microscopic: parallel bundles of fibrocytes often associated with lipocytes.
- Treatment: excision.

**4. Hidradenoma**

- Benign tumor of apocrine glands, occurs rarely in blacks.
- Can be misdiagnosed as adenocarcinoma.
- Gross: smaller than 2 cm in size arising from the labia majora or interlabial sulci.
- Microscopic: adenomatous pattern consisting of numerous tubules and acini lined with a layer of columnar cells (eosinophilic cytoplasm and vesicular nucleus) and a layer of myoepithelial cells.
- Treatment: excision and careful histologic evaluation.

**5. Schwannoma *(granular cell myoblastoma)***

- Tumor of nerve sheath.
- Microscopic
    - Irregular nests of large polyhedral cells whose cytoplasm is packed with numerous eosinophilic granules.
    - Overlying epidermis often exhibits pseudoepitheliomatous hyperplasia that mimics invasive squamous carcinoma.
- Treatment: large excision with free margins.

**6. Nevi**

- Gross: pigmented lesions in general; nevi may be nonpigmented.
- Microscopic: nests of nevus cells with round or ovoid nuclei, situated at the dermoepidermal junction (junctional nevi), the dermis (dermal) or both (compound).
- Treatment: excision for diagnosis (differential diagnosis with carcinoma in situ, melanoma, seborrheic keratosis).

7. **Seborrheic keratosis**
   - May mimic melanoma, nevi, or carcinoma in situ.
   - Gross: dark lesion, asymptomatic and with no malignant potential; brown lesion elsewhere on the body.
   - Microscopic: hyperkeratosis, acanthosis, papillomatosis, and horny keratin cysts.
   - Treatment: excision for diagnosis (no treatment necessary if the diagnosis is secure).
8. **Accessory breast**
   - Common along the embryologic "milk lines" (axillae, lower chest, upper abdomen), rare in vulva.
   - Enlargement of labia, in association with pregnancy.
   - High incidence of malignancy (4 cases of primary cancer of breast in vulva have been published).
   - Microscopic: identical to breast tissue, glandular acini and ducts.
   - Treatment: local excision (not during pregnancy).
9. **Endometrioma**
   - Due to implantation of endometrium at delivery or surgery.
   - Gross: bluish red cystic mass with cyclic enlargement.
   - Microscopic: endometrial glands and stroma.
   - Treatment: excision.
10. **Syringoma**
    - Gross: small asymptomatic skin-colored or yellow nodules on both labia majora.
    - Microscopic: dilated eccrine glands lined by

stratified epithelium with terminal comma-shaped tails.

- No treatment required.

## VII. Non-neoplastic epithelial disorders

- New classification (1987) by the International Society for the Study of Vulvar Diseases (ISSVD) and the International Society of Gynecological Pathologists (ISGP): lichen sclerosus, squamous hyperplasia, and other dermatoses.
- Old classification (1975): lichen sclerosus, hyperplastic dystrophy, mixed dystrophy.

### A. Lichen sclerosus

- Found in all age groups.
- Gross: thin, parchment-like whitish area.
- Microscopic: hyperkeratosis, thin epithelium, with loss of rete ridges, collagenized layer, inflammatory cells.
- Diagnosis by biopsy.
- Patients have low serum dihydrotestosterone and high free testosterone (Friedrich).
- Treatment: testosterone or progesterone creams.
- Incidence of malignancy: rare.

### B. Squamous hyperplasia *(equivalent to hyperplastic dystrophy)*

- Gross: thick white, red, or bright pink areas, sometimes cartilaginous.
- Microscopic: hyperkeratosis, acanthosis, with widening and clubbing of rete ridges, chronic inflammation.
- Diagnosis by biopsy, essentially diagnosis by exclusion.
- Treatment: topical corticosteroid.

- Incidence of malignancy: low in the presence of atypia (2–3%).

## VIII. Neoplastic intraepithelial disorders

### A. Definition of atypia in vulvar epithelium

1. **Pearl formation at the rete tips or in the basal layers.**
2. **Anaplastic, immature cells in the epithelium *(mitosis, high nucleocytoplasmic [N/C] ratio).***
3. **Corps ronds formation *(nuclear pycnosis with perinuclear halo).***

### B. Classification of vulvar epithelial neoplasia (VIN)

1. **VIN I (mild dysplasia):** atypia in lower ⅓ of the epithelium.
2. **VIN II (moderate dysplasia):** atypia in lower ⅔ of the epithelium.
3. **VIN III (severe dysplasia):** atypia in more than ⅔ of the epithelium.

### C. Types of intraepithelial neoplastic disorders of vulva

1. **Squamous cell carcinoma in situ (VIN III)**
   - Formerly called Bowen's disease, erythroplasia of Queyrat, carcinoma simplex.
   - Gross: single or multiple lesions, macular or papular. Variety of color: dark, white, gray, pink, or red.
   - Microscopic: hyperkeratosis, parakeratosis, abnormal cells in all layers of the epithelium (giant cells, corps ronds, mitoses, individual cell keratinization).
   - Treatment: wide local excision with clear margins; recurrences can be treated with 5FU

ointment (painful because of necrosis); skinning vulvectomy with split-thickness skin graft in case of multicentric lesions (DiSaia); destruction with hot cautery, laser surgery (pain, bleeding, infection, but cosmetic results excellent); cryosurgery (slow healing, pain).

- Progression to invasive carcinoma is rare (6%), and usually occurs in postmenopausal women.
- *Bowenoid papulosis*
  - Clinical entity described by Wade and Ackerman in 1978.
  - Seen in young patients (18–38 years), and in pregnant patients.
  - Asymptomatic or itching, burning, pain.
  - Gross: often multiple papules, 1–10 mm, reddish brown or pinkish.
  - Microscopic: hyperkeratosis, focal parakeratosis, dyskeratosis, large hyperchromatic pleomorphic nuclei of epidermal cells, atypical mitoses (similar to carcinoma in situ).
  - Natural history still unknown; spontaneous regression can occur. Its cause is thought to be viral (HPV 16).
  - Considered a form of carcinoma in situ (CIS) of vulva.
  - Treatment: excision or local destruction (laser).

**2. Paget's disease**

- Rare; 25% are invasive (75% remain intraepithelial); found in 6th–8th decades.
- Not always associated with an underlying adenocarcinoma (unlike Paget's disease of the nipple, which is always associated with duct carcinoma of breast); can be associated with

other malignancies: adnexal carcinoma of skin, cervix, breast, rectum.

- Gross: brick-red lesion with white islands.
- Microscopic: nests of Paget's cells (large cells with abundant finely granular and clear cytoplasm, basophilic nuclei) in the parabasal layer of the epithelium, involving the appendages in 75% of cases. Invasive disease may be demonstrated by direct invasion of the Paget's cells and undifferentiated basal cells into underlying stroma.
- Treatment: wide local excision of the lesion, including the underlying dermis to rule out adenocarcinoma (frozen section of surgical margins); in case of associated underlying adenocarcinoma, radical vulvectomy with groin lymph node dissection (prognosis guarded in case of positive nodes).
- Recurrences are frequent even when the margins are free.

## IX. Invasive malignancies

- Constitute 4% of all primary malignancies of the genital canal.
- FIGO clinical staging according to T (tumor), N (nodes), M (metastases). (FIGO [International Federation of Obstetricians and Gynecologists], 1988.)
  - *Stage I:* tumor confined to vulva and/or perineum, 2 cm or less in greatest dimension. No nodal metastasis.
  - *Stage II:* tumor confined to vulva and/or perineum, exceeding 2 cm in greatest diameter. No nodal metastasis.
  - *Stage III:* tumor of any size with adjacent spread to the lower urethra and/or the vagina, the anus, and/or unilateral regional lymph node metastasis.

- *Stage IVA:* tumor invades any of the following: upper urethra, bladder mucosa, rectal mucosa, pelvic bone, and/or bilateral regional node metastasis.
- *Stage IVB:* any distant metastasis, including pelvic lymph nodes.

## A. Microinvasive carcinoma (Figure 1)

- Poorly defined entity—findings in the cervix can't be extrapolated to the vulva.
- Depth of invasion 5 mm: 15.2% of patients have inguinal lymph node metastasis. Depth of invasion 3 mm: 12.1% of patients have inguinal lymph node metastasis (Wilkinson).
- Measurement of depth of invasion different from one study to another. No uniform, universally accepted definition of microinvasive carcinoma of vulva.

### 1. Woodruff (1981)

a. *Microinvasion* defined as nests of "invading cells" between but not beyond the tips of the papillary ridges—no lymph node metastasis. Treatment by wide local excision—no recurrence (13 cases).

b. *Early invasion* (measured from the basal layer of the deepest rete peg)

- Between 0.1 and 1 mm: 8 cases; 2 had recurrences and died of disease. (Less than 0.8 mm: no recurrence.)
- Between 1.1 and 4 mm: 27 cases; 3 died of disease.
- Best treatment at this time: wide local excision or simple vulvectomy with sampling of the nodes.

### 2. Wilkinson (1982)

- Measurement made from the basement membrane of the most superficial adjacent dermal papilla to the deepest point of invasion.

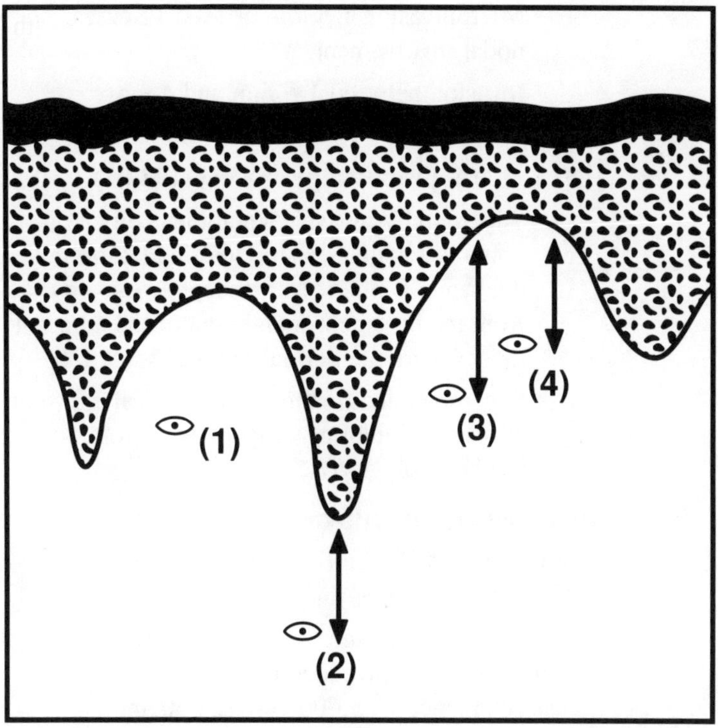


**Figure 1. Different concepts of microinvasive carcinoma of the vulva.**

(1) Woodruff: microinvasion (lesion between rete pegs).
(2) Woodruff: early invasion (lesion 0.1–1 mm from basal layer of deepest rete peg).
(3) Wilkinson: microinvasion (lesion 1.5 mm or less from basement membrane of most superficial adjacent dermal papilla).
(4) ISSVD: superficial invasion (lesion 1 mm from basement membrane of the most superficial adjacent dermal papilla).

- Microinvasion 1.5 mm or less: 12 cases, no nodal involvement.
- Invasion between 1.5 mm and 4 mm: 18 cases, 2 with node metastases (11%).

**3. Criteria proposed by ISSVD (1983)**

- Superficially invasive squamous cell carcinoma is a solitary lesion less than 2 cm in diameter; 1 mm or less in depth measured from the basement membrane of the adjacent most superficial dermal papilla (stage IA).
- Recommended treatment: wide local excision of lesion. Sampling of ipsilateral groin nodes has been suggested.

## B. Invasive squamous cell carcinoma

- Constitutes 90% of all vulvar malignancies, 4% of all female genital malignancies.
- Disease of the 7th and 8th decades; patients 20 years younger if preceded by granulomatous disease (incidence 1/25,000 between 60 and 70 years, 1.5/100,000 all women).
- Precursors: squamous hyperplasia with atypia, granulomatous disease, long-standing pruritus (more than 5 years).
- Most common site: upper labia majora.
- Gross: three-dimensional growth—⅓ are endophytic and ulcerated, ⅔ are exophytic and nodular or vegetative.
- Lymphatic invasion: superficial inguinal ("sentinel nodes"—DiSaia) and femoral nodes first, then deep femoral, then pelvic nodes. Incidence of lymph node involvement: for lesion less than 2 cm, 20%; for lesion more than 2 cm, 45% (Morley).
- Pathology:
  - Well-differentiated keratinizing carcinoma: 75% of lesions, large anastomosing masses of atypi-

cal squamous epithelium with nests of keratin (pearls) in the stroma.

- Poorly differentiated epidermoid tumors: 20% of lesions, nuclear polymorphism with numerous mitoses and minimal keratin formation.

- Survival is not influenced by degree of differentiation of the tumor.
- Treatment: radical vulvectomy with bilateral inguinal and femoral lymphadenectomy, may be altered if lesion is unilateral. If inguinal nodes are involved, irradiation of pelvic nodes is suggested.
- Five-year survival: 70%.
  - Stages I and II without node involvement: 90%.
  - Stages I and II with node involvement: 40%.
  - Five-year survival with positive pelvic nodes: 7% (Morley).

## C. Verrucous carcinoma

- Also called giant condyloma of Buschke and Lowenstein.
- Gross lesions mimic condyloma acuminata, locally invasive and recurrent with no involvement of the lymph nodes.
- Biopsy should be deep with large amount of stroma for pathologic diagnosis.
- Histology: papillary fronds of mature stratified squamous epithelium with bulbous rete pegs pushing the stroma. Hyperkeratosis and acanthosis. Uniform absence of malignant features such as nuclear anaplasia except occasional pearl formation in the epithelium but not at rete tips. Stroma infiltrated by inflammatory cells.
- Treatment: wide local excision with tumor-free margins. No lymph node metastasis in 27 cases (Japaze et al).
- Radiotherapy contraindicated because of possi-

bility of anaplastic transformation of benign to malignant cells.

## D. Adenocarcinoma

- Rarest of vulvar malignancies.
- Arises as primary tumor of Bartholin's glands. Can arise from ectopic breast.
- Average age: one decade younger than women with epidermoid cancer of vulva.
- Microscopic: adenocarcinoma often poorly differentiated.
- Diagnosis often late because of frequent inflammations in that area (biopsy, if patient is more than 40 years old and has inflammation of Bartholin's glands).
- Treatment: radical vulvectomy with bilateral inguinal and femoral node dissection.
- Survival determined by stage at diagnosis.

## E. Adenoid cystic carcinoma

- Classic adenocarcinoma of the Bartholin glands, similar to the tumor in salivary glands. (Half of Bartholin's gland carcinomas are squamous.)
- Pathology: nests of cells with round, oval hyperchromatic nuclei and scant cytoplasm, arranged concentrically in a cribriform pattern around a gland-like space.
- Invades deeply, recurs locally, and metastasizes late, often to the lungs, rarely to groin nodes.
- Treatment: wide local excision with ipsilateral inguinal lymphadenectomy (Copeland et al).

## F. Basal cell carcinoma

- Constitutes 2% of vulvar cancers.
- Gross: ulcerative lesion with rolled, raised edges less than 2 cm in diameter.

- Microscopic: masses of small basal cells with monotonous pattern and palisading at the periphery.
- Metastasis to lymph node rare (one case reported).
- Treatment: wide local excision.

## G. Malignant melanoma

- Constitutes 2–3% of vulvar neoplasms.
- Gross pattern: elevated, pigmented, and frequently ulcerated growths. Two basic types: nodular and superficial spreading.
- Microscopic: bizarre, atypical melanocytes with junctional activity, prominent melanin pigmentation, deep invasion of the surrounding tissue, and abnormal mitotic figures. Great microscopic variability. Often misdiagnosed as undifferentiated squamous cancer.
- Clark's levels: I, intraepithelial; II, papillary dermis; III, interface papillary dermis and reticular dermis; IV, reticular dermis; and V, subcutaneous fat.
- Breslow's depth of invasion: low risk, less than 0.76 mm; intermediate, between 0.76 and 1.5 mm; high risk, greater than 1.5 mm.
- Treatment: radical vulvectomy, bilateral inguinal and femoral lymphadenectomy for those invading beyond Clark's level III; adjunctive chemotherapy with dacarbazine.
- Prognosis depends on the level of involvement (I, 100% 5-year survival; II, 100%; III, 74%; IV, 50%; V, 30%) and lymph node metastasis.
- Death with widespread metastases: lungs, liver, brain.

## H. Sarcomas

- Rare: 2% of vulvar cancers.
- Younger group of patients (mean age 38 years).

- Fibrosarcoma, rhabdomyosarcoma, neurofibrosarcoma, leiomyosarcoma (most common).
- Tend to recur locally.
- Treatment: radical vulvectomy and bilateral inguinal lymphadenectomy.
- Poor survival.

### I. Secondary malignant tumors

- Metastases from cervix, rectum, endometrium.
- Choriocarcinoma and hypernephroma.
- Malignant lymphoma.

## Suggested Readings

1. Boyce J, Fruchter RG, Kasambilides E, Nicastri AD, Sedlis A, Remy JC. Prognostic factors in carcinoma of the vulva. *Gynecol Oncol* 20:364, 1985.
2. Breen JL, Smith CI, Gregori CA. Extramammary Paget's Disease. *Clin Obstet Gynecol* 21:1107, 1978.
3. Buckley CH, Butler EB, Fox H. Vulvar intraepithelial neoplasia and microinvasive carcinoma of the vulva. *J Clin Pathol* 37:1201, 1984.
4. Butler EB, Stanbridge CM. Condylomatous lesions of the lower female genital tract. *Clin Obstet Gynecol* 11:171, 1984.
5. Copeland LJ, Sneige N, Gershenson DM, Saul PB, Stringer CA, Seski JC. Adenoid cystic carcinoma of Bartholin's gland. *Obstet Gynecol* 67:115, 1986.
6. DiSaia P. Management of superficially invasive vulvar carcinoma. *Clin Obstet Gynecol* 28:196, 1985.
7. Friedrich EG Jr. Vulvar dystrophy. *Clin Obstet Gynecol* 28:178, 1985.
8. Friedrich EG, Wilkinson EJ, Fu YS. Carcinoma in situ of the vulva: A continuing challenge. *Am J Obstet Gynecol* 136:830, 1980.
9. Hacker NF, Berek JS, Lagasse LD, Leuchter RS, Moore JG. Management of regional lymph nodes and their

prognostic influence in vulvar cancer. *Obstet Gynecol* 61:408, 1983.

10. Hacker NF, Berek JS, Lagasse LD, Nieberg RK, Leuchter RS. Individualization of treatment for stage I squamous cell vulvar carcinoma. *Obstet Gynecol* 63:155, 1984.
11. Jamarillo BA, Ganjei P, Averette HE, Sevin BU, Lovecchio JL. Malignant melanoma of the vulva. *Obstet Gynecol* 66:398, 1985.
12. Japaze H, Dinh TV, Woodruff JD. Verrucous carcinoma of the vulva: Study of 24 cases. *Obstet Gynecol* 60:462, 1982.
13. Kaufman RH, Bornstein J, Adam E, et al. Human papillomavirus and herpes simplex virus in vulvar squamous cell carcinoma in situ. *Am J Obstet Gynecol* 158:862, 1988.
14. Kaufman RH, Faro S. Herpes genitalis: Clinical features and treatment. *Clin Obstet Gynecol* 28:152, 1985.
15. Lynch PJ. Condylomata acuminata (anogenital warts). *Clin Obstet Gynecol* 28:142, 1985.
16. Parmley TH, Woodruff JD, Julian CG. Invasive vulvar Paget's disease. *Obstet Gynecol* 46:341, 1975.
17. Powell LC, Dinh TV, Rajaraman S, Hannigan EV, Dillard EA, Yandell RE, To T. Carcinoma in situ of the vulva: A clinicopathologic study of 50 cases. *J Reprod Med* 31:808, 1986.
18. Wilkinson EJ, Rico MJ, Pierson KK. Microinvasive carcinoma of the vulva. *Int J Gynecol Pathol* 1:29, 1982.
19. Woodruff JD, Friedrich EG. The vestibule. *Clin Obstet Gynecol* 28:134, 1985.

# 2. The Urethra

I. Embryology
II. Histology
III. Infections
IV. Benign tumors
V. Malignant tumors

## I. Embryology

- Epithelium is derived from the endodermal vesical part of the urogenital sinus. A portion may be derived from mesoderm of the mesonephric duct, thus may respond to estrogenic hormones.
- Connective tissue and smooth muscle develop from the adjacent splanchnic mesoderm.
- Paraurethral and suburethral glands (analogue to prostate) are outbuddings from the epithelium of the cranial part of the urethra.

## II. Histology

- Canal lined by transitional epithelium with stratified squamous epithelium at the orifice.
- Muscularis composed of longitudinal inner layer and circular outer layer of smooth muscle.

## III. Infections

### A. Infection of paraurethral ducts *(Skene's ducts)*

- Skene's ducts recognized at the posterior aspect of the external urethral meatus (orifice: squamous, duct: transitional epithelium).
- Orifice red, edematous, everted.
- Agents: gonococcus, Trichomonas.
- Treatment: antibiotics and metronidazole.

### B. Infection of suburethral glands

- Gross: suburethral diverticula resulting from recurrent chronic infection.
- Microscopic: chronic inflammation.
- Treatment: antibiotics, surgical excision of diverticula.

### C. Urethritis cystica

- Related to inflammation.
- Microscopic: small inclusions of transitional epithelium surrounded by chronically infected mucosa.

### D. Eversion of urethral meatus

- Occurs in prepubertal girls or postmenopausal women, due to atrophy of the adjacent mucosa.
- Reddened eversion of the urethral tissue, can be mistaken for a caruncle or other tumor.
- Treated locally with estrogens.

## IV. Benign tumors

### A. Caruncle

- Most common tumor.
- Gross: reddish, tender, polypoid lesion at the meatus.
- Microscopic: 3 forms—papillomatous, angiomatous, and granulomatous (small vessels surrounded by edematous stroma infiltrated with inflammatory cells).
- Treatment: excision for pathologic examination (to rule out urethral carcinoma).

### B. Condyloma acuminata, squamous papilloma: biopsy in case of doubt about the type of tumor.

## V. Malignant tumors

**A. Squamous carcinoma:** more common than other types.

**B. Transitional cell carcinoma, urethral variety:** similar to papillary carcinoma of the bladder.

**C. Adenocarcinoma:** rare, arising from the mucus-secreting glands of the suburethral area.

- Treatment for A, B, and C: interstitial irradiation to central lesion; inguinal lymphadenectomy followed by pelvic and local irradiation if inguinal nodes are positive.

**D. Sarcoma, melanoma, lymphoma:** usually secondary, very rare.

**E. Metastases from carcinoma of bladder, vulva, vagina, cervix, ovary, and choriocarcinoma.**

## Suggested Readings

1. Bolduan JP, Farah RN. Primary urethral neoplasms: Review of 30 cases. *J. Urol* 125:198, 1981.
2. Turner AG, Hendry WF. Primary carcinoma of the female urethra. *Br J Urol* 52:549, 1980.
3. Weghaupt K, Gerstner GJ, Kucera H. Radiation therapy for primary carcinoma of the female urethra: A survey over 25 years. *Gynecol Oncol* 17:58, 1984.
4. Zaino RJ. Carcinoma of vulva, urethra and Bartholin's gland. In: Contemporary issues in surgical pathology. *Pathology of the Vulva and Vagina* 9:119, 1987, New York, Churchill Livingstone.

# 3. The Vagina

I. Embryology
II. Histology
III. Inflammatory lesions
IV. Benign tumors
V. Malignancies

## I. Embryology

- Still in dispute, but most agree of mesodermal origin.
- Classic view:
  - Upper ⅓ results from fusion of the inferior portions of the müllerian ducts (mesoderm).
  - Lower ⅔ comes from canalization of a portion of the endoderm of the urogenital sinus.
- Recent studies (Forsberg): mesonephric ducts (wolffian ducts) involved in the formation of the vaginal plate (intermediate zone between the müllerian ducts and the urogenital sinus). The vaginal epithelium is then derived from two sources, both mesodermal:
  - Upper ⅓ is derived from fused müllerian ducts.
  - Lower ⅔ is derived from vaginal plate, which is formed by proliferation of cells from the patch of mesodermal epithelium derived from the wolffian ducts. It is situated in the posterior wall of the urogenital sinus between the orifices of the two

wolffian ducts and the point at which the fused müllerian ducts abut (Parmley).

## II. Histology

- Epithelium: nonkeratinizing stratified squamous epithelium composed of superficial, intermediate, parabasal, and basal cells; responds to hormones.
- Lamina propria (stroma), with mesonephric remnants in the fornices.
- Maturation index: ratio of percentages of parabasal/intermediate/superficial cells (birth 0-95-5, childhood 80-20-0, ovulation 0-40-60, pregnancy 0-95-5, postpartum 100-0-0, menopause 100-0-0).

## III. Inflammatory lesions

### A. Bacterial, protozoa, and fungal agents:

Trichomonas vaginalis (treatment: metronidazole). Monilia (treatment: imidazoles). Leptothrix, Gardnerella vaginalis (treatment: metronidazole, cephradine). Actinomyces israelii (treatment: penicillin).

**B. Herpes:** cytologic findings and culture as in vulva.

### C. Vaginitis emphysematosa

- Numerous small cysts lined by a syncytium of foreign body giant cells.
- No specific bacteria, but Trichomonas commonly associated with it.
- Found in pregnancy and in heart failure.
- Condition disappears after treatment of trichomoniasis.

### D. Vaginitis in children

- Gonococcal, very persistent infection.
- Foreign bodies.

### E. Vaginitis, postmenopausal

- Vagina thin: bleeding, burning, dyspareunia.
- Histology: thin epithelium without surface maturation, nonspecific inflammation in the stroma.
- Treatment: estrogens.

**F. Syphilis:** chancre diagnosed by dark field microscopy, biopsy, and special stain.

### G. Granulation tissue

- Common at the apex of the vault, after hysterectomy.
- To be differentiated from prolapsed tubal fimbria after hysterectomy.

### H. Tampon ulcer

- Associated with the use of superabsorbent tampons.
- Gross: mucosa red or ulcerated.
- Microscopic: ulceration of epithelium replaced by granulation tissue. Foreign body may be found in biopsy.
- No treatment needed. Ulcers will heal after discontinuing the use of tampons.

## IV. Benign tumors

### A. Gartner's duct cysts

- Remnants of the wolffian ducts.
- Found in the anterolateral position of the vaginal wall.
- Microscopic: epithelium lined by a single layer of low cuboidal epithelium. Squamous metaplasia not uncommon.
- Treatment: excision if large.

## B. Vaginal inclusion cysts.

- Found in the posterior or lateral wall of the vagina.
- Due to inclusion of the vaginal epithelium during surgery.
- Microscopic: cyst lined by squamous epithelium.
- Treatment: excision if large.

## C. Mucinous cysts

- Remnants of the incomplete separation of the rectum and urogenital sinus by the urorectal fold.
- Treatment: excision if large.

## D. Endometriosis

- Common site: posterior fornix.
- Microscopic: endometrial glands and stroma.
- Treatment: excision if large.

## E. Adenosis

- Common complaint: excess mucous discharge.
- Partial conversion of the squamous vaginal epithelium to glandular epithelium of endocervical type.
- Gross: pebbly, red granular patches not stained with iodine or colposcopically abnormal, frequently at upper third of vagina, on anterior wall.
- Microscopic: mucin-producing columnar glands similar to those of endocervix; sometimes dark and light, ciliated cells resembling the lining of endometrium or fallopian tube (20% of specimens). Areas of adenosis can undergo squamous metaplasia (as in cervix), microglandular hyperplasia (with oral contraceptive agents), Arias-Stella phenomenon.
- Tubal-endometrial form of adenosis occurs more often with clear cell adenocarcinoma.

- Among patients exposed in utero to diethylstilbestrol (DES) during their first 8 weeks of life, 90% have adenosis; among those exposed after the 16th week, 10% have adenosis.
- Often associated with transverse or concentric vaginal ridges, or with cockscomb of cervix.
- Potential for developing cancer is small (0.14/1000 to 1.4/1000 DES-exposed daughters).
- Adenosis is common and found at autopsy in 40% of patients who have no gross abnormalities but who have had serial sections of the vagina (Sandberg).
- No treatment.
- Follow patient every year.

### F. Condyloma acuminatum *(similar to lesions found on vulva and cervix).*

### G. Leiomyoma

- Most common benign tumor.
- Microscopic: interlacing bundles of spindle-shaped smooth muscle cells.
- Treatment: excision if large.

### H. Vaginal polyp

- Gross: single or multiple finger-like projections.
- Microscopic: loose, edematous stroma with atypical cells can simulate sarcoma botryoides (but with no hypercellular cambium layer).
- Treatment: local excision curative.

### I. Prolapsed fallopian tube

- Rare complication of vaginal and abdominal surgery.
- Gross: small bleeding mass at apex of vulva, biopsy painful.

- Microscopic: tubal mucosa with inflammatory cells in stroma.
- Treatment: excision.

# V. Malignancies

## A. Carcinoma in situ

- Gross: whitish, hyperkeratotic and erythroplastic foci, multifocal lesions in the upper third of the vagina.
- Microscopic: full thickness alterations in maturation of the epithelium (immature cells, loss of polarity, high N/C ratio, atypical mitoses).
- Treatment: wide local excision, 5FU cream (2% or 5%), laser.

## B. Invasive epidermoid carcinoma of the vagina

- Constitutes 0.5% of all primary genital canal malignancies.
- Common site: upper ⅓ of vagina anterior and posterior walls.
- Lymphatic extension
  - Upper ⅔: pelvic nodes (as in cervix).
  - Lower ⅓: inguinal and femoral nodes (as in vulva).
- FIGO staging:
  - *Stage 0:* intraepithelial.
  - *Stage I:* limited to vaginal wall.
  - *Stage II:* subvaginal tissue.
  - *Stage III:* extension to pelvic wall.
  - *Stage IV:* beyond true pelvis, into bladder or rectum.
- Gross: nodular or ulcerative lesions.

- Microscopic: epidermoid type with various degrees of maturation.
- Treatment: radiotherapy (external irradiation and radium applications); surgery (radical hysterectomy, vaginectomy, and pelvic lymphadenectomy) in selected patients.
- Five-year survival: for stage I, 73%; for all stages, 51%.

## C. Adenocarcinoma of vagina

- Rare.
- Arises in young women (7–29 years) whose mothers received DES during pregnancy (500 cases of clear cell adenocarcinoma of vagina and cervix reported to 1986).
- Incidence of malignancy 1/1000 to 1/10,000 in DES-exposed females.
- Median age at time of diagnosis: 19 years.
- Gross: tumor at cervix (40%) or anterior wall of upper third of vagina (60%).
- Microscopic: tubules and cysts lined by clear cells and hobnail cells (mesonephroma), or sheets of clear cells. Tubopapillary form is said to be most aggressive.
- Treatment: surgery (radical excision of vagina and uterus and pelvic lymphadenectomy) or irradiation.
- Overall 5-year survival: 80%.

## D. Melanoma

- Rare.
- Predilection for anterior wall and distal third of vagina.
- Treatment: radical surgery.
- Prognostic poor (overall survival 14%) because diagnosis is usually late (level III).

## E. Fibrosarcoma or leiomyosarcoma

- Rare.
- Gross: solitary mass in the anterior and lateral vaginal walls.
- Microscopic: more than 5 mitoses per high power fields (HPF) and significant cellular atypia (Tavassoli and Norris).
- Patients over 50 years old: more aggressive course.
- Treatment: surgery (local excision).

## F. Sarcoma botryoides

- Rare, usually occurs in girls under 5 years old.
- Symptoms: vaginal bleeding and discharge.
- Gross: edematous, grayish red polypoid masses filling the vagina.
- Microscopic: extensive edema of stroma, crowding of cells under the epithelium (cambium layer of Nicholson), rhabdomyoblasts—can be misinterpreted as a benign polyp.
- Treatment: surgical resection of gross disease followed by adjuvant chemotherapy (vincristine, actinomycin D, and cyclophosphamide—VAC; or VAC plus Adriamycin) with or without radiation.
- Survival 3 years: 78% (Copeland et al).

## G. Endodermal sinus tumor

- Very rare.
- Grossly simulates sarcoma botryoides.
- Microscopic: like ovarian counterpart; loose vacuolated network with Schiller-Duval bodies.
- Treatment: surgery and triple chemotherapy (VAC). Prognosis improved with chemotherapy.
- Survival 3 years: 84% (with chemotherapy).

### H. Metastatic carcinomas

1. **Cervix, endometrium.**
2. **Rectum, bladder.**
3. **Choriocarcinoma**
   - Gross: dark blue hemorrhagic nodule.
   - Microscopic: trophoblastic tissue (cytotrophoblast and syncytiotrophoblast).
   - Treatment: chemotherapy (80% cure rate).

## Suggested Readings


1. Copeland LJ, Gershenson DM, Saul PB, et al. Sarcoma botryoides of the female genital tract. *Obstet Gynecol* 66:262, 1985.
2. Forsberg JG. Cervicovaginal epithelium: Its origin and development. *Am J Obstet Gynecol* 115:1025, 1973.
3. Friedrich EG, Siegesmund KA. Tampon associated vaginal ulcerations. *Obstet Gynecol* 55:149, 1980.
4. Herbst AL, Ulfelder H, Poskanzer DC. Adenocarcinoma of the vagina: Association of maternal stilbestrol therapy with tumor appearance in young women. *N Eng J Med* 284:878, 1971.
5. Jefferies JA, Robboy SJ, O'Brien PC, et al. Structural anomalies of the cervix and vagina in women enrolled in the diethylstilbestrol adenosis (DESAD) project. *Am J Obstet Gynecol* 148:59, 1984.
6. Miettinen M, Wahlstrom T, Vesterinen E, et al. Vaginal polyps with pseudosarcomatous features: A clinicopathologic study of seven cases. *Cancer* 51:1148, 1983.
7. Parmley T. Embryology of the female genital tract. In: Kurman RJ (ed). *Blaustein's pathology of the female genital tract*. 3d ed. New York: Springer-Verlag, 1987.
8. Petrilli ES, Townsend DE, Morrow CP, et al. Vaginal intraepithelial neoplasia: Biologic aspects and treatment with topical 5-Fluorouracil and the carbon dioxide laser. *Am J Obstet Gynecol* 138:321, 1980.

9. Robboy SJ, Hill EC, Sandberg EC, Czernobilsky B. Vaginal adenosis in women born prior to the diethylstilbestrol (DES) era. *Hum Pathol* 17:488, 1986.
10. Sandberg EC. The incidence and distribution of occult vaginal adenosis. *Am J Obstet Gynecol* 101:322, 1968.
11. Tavassoli FA, Norris HJ. Smooth muscle tumors of the vagina. *Obstet Gynecol* 53:689, 1979.

# 4. The Cervix


I. Embryology
II. Histology
III. Cervical changes in pregnancy
IV. Squamous metaplasia
V. Koilocytotic atypia
VI. Inflammations
VII. Benign lesions
VIII. Malignant tumors


## I. Embryology

- Cervix is of mesodermal origin.
- Results from fusion of the middle portions of müllerian ducts.
- Adjacent mesenchyme gives rise to stroma and muscle fibers.
- Stratified squamous and columnar epitheliums are derived from the epithelium of the primitive mesoderm.

## II. Histology

**A. Exocervix:** nonkeratinizing stratified squamous epithelium (no cornification, unless cervix is prolapsed) composed of superficial, intermediate, and parabasal cells.

**B. Endocervix:** columnar epithelium composed of cylindrical "picket-fence," mucus-secreting cells with basally placed nuclei. Reserve cells under the columnar epithelium.

**C. Stroma:** spindle cells with decidual reaction during pregnancy; contains (1%) cystic remnants of mesonephric ducts (which can have adenomatous patterns).

## III. Cervical changes in pregnancy

### A. Exocervix

- Increase in thickness, cellular abnormalities in the basal layers suggesting dysplasia.
- These changes regress after pregnancy and should be carefully evaluated in order to avoid an error in diagnosis.

### B. Endocervix

- Glandular hyperplasia: increase in the number of glands with adenomatous pattern and secretory overactivity.
- Glandular epithelial hyperplasia: pile up into 2 to 3 layers.
- Squamous and mucoid metaplasia.
- Arias-Stella reaction cells with hyperchromatic nuclei suggesting malignancy; no mitoses.

**C. Stroma:** increase in vascularity (cuffing of small arteries), edema, leucocytic infiltration (50%), decidual reaction (10%).

## IV. Squamous metaplasia

- Replacement of the mucus-secreting glandular epithelium of the endocervix by stratified squamous epithelium.
- Characterized by proliferation and metaplasia of the

reserve or indifferent cells, under the columnar epithelium.

- Constitutes the pattern at the transitional zone of the cervix (T-zone), which is also the site of cervical epidermoid neoplasia.
- Can give confusing pictures that lead to an erroneous diagnosis of carcinoma.

## V. Koilocytotic atypia

- Found in condyloma acuminata which can be papillomatous (classic), flat, or inverted in the cervix.
- Composed of cells with hyperchromatic, irregular, pycnotic, sometimes double nuclei, and with perinuclear clearing of the cytoplasm ("balloon cells").
- Evidence of papilloma virus infection which should be identified by hybridization.
- Can be found in cervical intraepithelial neoplasia (CIN) lesions.
- Treatment: according to the degree of dysplasia.

## VI. Inflammations

### A. Chronic cervicitis

- Gross: everted endocervix, hyperemic and edematous mucosa, Nabothian cysts.
- Microscopic: subepithelial inflammatory infiltrate (plasma cells, polymorphonuclear leucocytes, monocytes), frequent diagnosis.
- Treatment: no need for therapy.

### B. Tuberculous cervicitis

- Rare, often secondary to tuberculous salpingitis and endometritis or tuberculosis in consort.

- Gross: ulceration or hypertrophic lesion that simulates carcinoma.
- Microscopic: classic tubercle with lymphocytes, epithelioid cells, giant cells and central caseation; identification of specific bacillus.
- Treatment: antituberculosis drugs.

### C. Actinomycosis

- Caused by Actinomyces israelii, a gram-positive anaerobe.
- Associated with intrauterine devices (IUD).
- Microscopic: granules composed of branching, gram-positive filaments with peripheral palisading clubs, identified by silver stain.
- Treatment: penicillin.

### D. Condylomata acuminata

- Microscopic: papillomatosis, parakeratosis, koilocytosis, inflammatory infiltrate in stroma.
- Treatment: trichloracetic acid, electrocautery, laser.

### E. Herpes

- Microscopic: multinucleated squamous cells with intranuclear "ground glass" viral eosinophilic inclusions.
- Treatment: acyclovir.

### F. Chlamydia trachomatis

- Mucopurulent cervicitis (yellow-green exudate).
- Often associated with follicular cervicitis.
- Diagnosis by culture.
- Treatment: tetracycline, doxycycline, erythromycin.

# VII. Benign lesions

## A. Endocervical polyp

- Gross: localized proliferation of cervical mucosa as a bright red, vascular, pedunculated fragile growth.
- Microscopic: polyp lined by endocervical epithelium or stratified squamous epithelium; stroma loose, edematous with inflammatory infiltrate.
- Clinical: bleeding due to vascularity and infection, simulates early carcinoma.
- Rarely become malignant (0.2–0.4%).
- To be differentiated from a polypoid carcinoma (pedicle *not* invaded by carcinoma in secondary malignancy in a polyp).
- Treatment: excision for pathologic examination.

## B. Nabothian cyst

- Mucous retention cyst due to coverage by squamous epithelium of an endocervical cleft.
- Variable size (3 mm to 3 cm), lined by columnar or flat epithelium.
- Generally asymptomatic, no treatment required.

## C. Endometriosis

- Gross: bluish nodule.
- Microscopic: endometrial glands with stroma.
- Treatment: biopsy for diagnosis.

## D. Leiomyoma

- Posterior cervix.
- Microscopic: interlacing bundles of smooth muscle cells.
- Treatment: myomectomy or hysterectomy because of frequent association of cervical with uterine leiomyoma.

### E. Adenomas or cysts due to vestiges of mesonephric ducts

- Lined by a low columnar or cuboidal epithelium.
- May be confused with adenocarcinoma.
- Treatment: excision if large.

### F. Microglandular hyperplasia *(microcystic mucoid hyperplasia)*

- Resembles polyps 1–2 cm in size.
- Occurs during use of oral contraceptive agents (OCA) or during prolonged estrogen therapy, or during pregnancy.
- Can be mistaken for adenocarcinoma.
- Microscopic: complex proliferation of tightly packed small glands lined by flattened or cuboidal epithelial cells with no nuclear atypia; mucoid infiltration of the stroma with chronic inflammation.
- No treatment required.

### G. Adenosis

- Cockscomb (hood), collar (rim), or pseudopolyp of cervix.
- Found in DES daughters.
- Ectropion and squamous metaplasia are frequent.
- Microscopic: analogous to adenosis of vagina.
- No treatment required.

## VIII. Malignant tumors

### A. Malignant changes in cervix: cervical intra-epithelial neoplasia *(CIN—Richart)*

- Disarray and loss of polarity of different layers of the epithelium.
- Cellular anaplasia; loss of normal maturation: attempted keratinization in deeper layers, para-

basal type cells in upper layers, bizarre nuclear figures, abnormal mitoses.

1. **CIN I (mild dysplasia):** neoplastic cells with mitoses extend to ⅓ of the thickness of the epithelium.
2. **CIN II (moderate dysplasia):** cellular aberrations extend to ⅔ of the thickness of the epithelium.
3. **CIN III (severe dysplasia and carcinoma in situ):** cellular aberrations extend to more than ⅔ of the thickness of the epithelium.
    - Mean transition time from CIN I and CIN II to CIN III is approximately 5.8 years and 3.1 years respectively. Mean transition time from CIN III to invasive carcinoma is 10 years (Richart and Barron).
    - Treatment: cryocautery, electrocautery, laser, or conization, after colposcopy and endocervical curettage.

## B. Microinvasive carcinoma (Figure 2)

- Constitutes 4% of all CIN.
- Depth of stromal invasion should be measured on a conization or a hysterectomy specimen.
- Depth of stromal invasion: 3 mm (Gynecologic Oncology Group [GOG]) or 5 mm (FIGO) from the basement membrane; no confluence of invasive foci and no vascular permeation.
- New definition of FIGO adds 7 mm of horizontal spread.
- Measurement from basement membrane of adjacent surface epithelium or "glandular" epithelium.
- Positive pelvic nodes 8% if stromal invasion is 3–5 mm, 0.2% if invasion 1–3 mm (1–5 mm depth of invasion: 1.8% node metastasis).

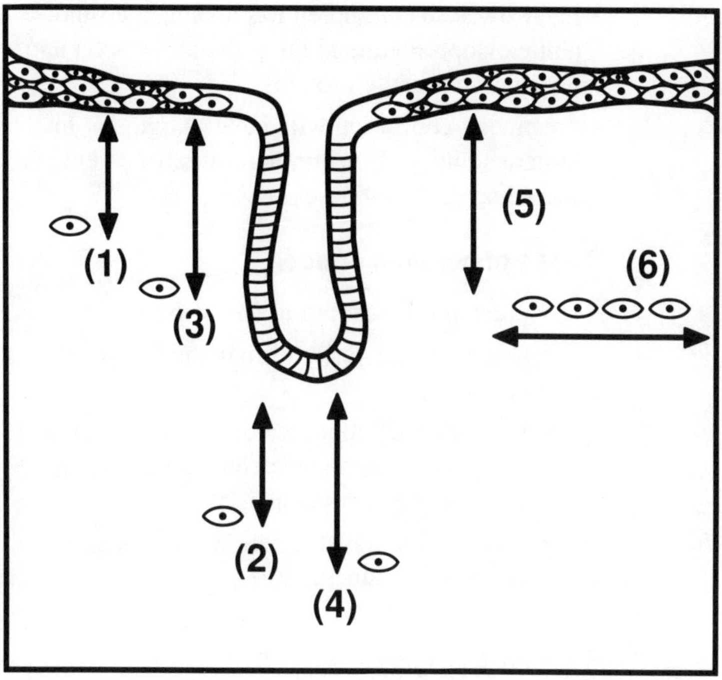


**Figure 2. Different concepts of microinvasive carcinoma of the cervix.**

(1, 2) GOG: 3 mm from basement membrane of surface epithelium or "glandular" epithelium (endocervical cleft).

(3, 4) FIGO: 5 mm from basement membrane of surface epithelium or "glandular" epithelium.

(5, 6) New FIGO stage $IA_2$: 5 mm in depth from basement membrane of surface epithelium or "glandular" epithelium and 7 mm in width.

- Early invasive cancer cell has abundant eosinophilic cytoplasm due to the presence of actin and myosin (contractile proteins).
- Treatment: conization with clear margins or total hysterectomy (only with microinvasive carcinoma according to definition of GOG).

## C. Types of cervical cancer

### 1. Epidermoid carcinoma (most frequent)

- Constitutes majority of malignancies of cervix (90%).
- May be exophytic, ulcerative, or infiltrating (exophytic lesion can create barrel-shaped lesion in the cervical canal).
- Arises at the transformation zone (or squamocolumnar junction).
- Sites: anterior and posterior lips (60–75%).
- FIGO staging
  - *Stage 0:* intraepithelial carcinoma (CIS).
  - *Stage I:* strictly confined to cervix.
    - *IA.* early stromal invasion.
      - *$IA_1$:* minimal microscopic stromal invasion.
      - *$IA_2$:* depth of invasion $\leq$ 5 mm, horizontal spread $\leq$ 7 mm.
    - *IB:* all other lesions greater than $IA_2$, whether seen clinically or not.
  - *Stage II:* extends beyond the cervix but has not extended onto the pelvic wall. Involves the vagina but not the lower ⅓.
    - *IIA:* vagina with no obvious parametrial involvement.
    - *IIB:* obvious parametrial involvement.
  - *Stage III:* may extend onto the pelvic wall. Involves the lower ⅓ of vagina.

- *IIIA:* no extension onto the pelvic wall; involvement of the lower ⅓ of vagina.
- *IIIB:* extension onto the pelvic wall; hydronephrosis or a nonfunctioning kidney.

- *Stage IV:* extension outside the reproductive tract. Involves the mucosa of the bladder or rectum, distant metastases.
  - *IVA:* adjacent organs (mucosa of bladder or rectum).
  - *IVB:* distant organs.

- Histologic classification based on degree of differentiation of tumor.
  - Well-differentiated, moderately differentiated (most frequent), and poorly differentiated

  or

  - Large-cell-keratinizing, large-cell-nonkeratinizing (best prognosis), and small-cell-nonkeratinizing (worse prognosis) (Reagan and Ng).
- Microscopic: interanastomosing tongues or solid masses of malignant cells infiltrating the stroma.
  - Well-differentiated (grade I): abundance of keratin formation (keratin pearls); cells mature and voluminous with large, hyperchromatic nuclei; mitoses; stroma infiltrated by chronic inflammatory cells and occasionally foreign body giant cells.
  - Moderately differentiated (grade II): neoplastic cells are more pleomorphic with large irregular nuclei and less abundant cytoplasm. Keratin pearls absent. Mitoses more abundant.
  - Poorly differentiated (grade III): cells

with hyperchromatic oval nuclei and scant indistinct cytoplasm. Sometimes large pleomorphic cells with bizarre nuclei and abnormal mitoses.

- Prognosis depends on clinical stage and tumor mass, not on cell type, except the small cell with neurosecretory granules.
- Lymphatic spread: paracervical, hypogastric, external iliac nodes.
- Clinical
  - Symptoms: bleeding after intercourse, bloody malodorous discharge.
  - Treatment
    - Stages IB and IIA: radical hysterectomy and pelvic lymphadenectomy or irradiation (barrel-shaped lesion: irradiation and extrafacial hysterectomy).
    - Stages IIB, III, IV: irradiation.
  - Node involvement: stage I, 15%; stage II, 30%; stage III, 50%.
  - Five-year survival: stage I, 85%; stage II, 60%; stage III, 35%; stage IV, 15%.

**2. Adenocarcinoma**

- Constitutes 5% of all carcinomas of cervix. Recent increase due to reduction in epidermoid cancer or increase in adenocarcinoma?
- Gross: papillary or ulcerative lesion in the cervical canal or in the region of the external os; bulky neoplasm which expands the endocervical canal (barrel-shaped lesion).

a. *In situ adenocarcinoma:* diagnosis made on conization or hysterectomy specimens—normal endocervical "glands" admixed with neoplastic glands, the cells of which show loss of polarity, enlargement and hyperchromatism of nuclei, and mitoses. Absence of stromal response. Can be confused with inflammation, Arias Stella reaction, and microcystic mucoid metaplasia. Often associated with epidermoid CIS. Treatment: simple hysterectomy or conization with free margins.

- Microinvasive adenocarcinoma is not an acceptable diagnosis.

b. *Endocervical adenocarcinoma*

- Closely packed glands that eliminate the stroma, cells with increased N/C ratio.
- Grades: I, II, III: well-differentiated, moderately differentiated (most common), and poorly differentiated. Extremely well differentiated lesion is called adenoma malignum or minimal deviation adenocarcinoma, difficult to recognize, and often associated with Peutz-Jeghers syndrome.
- If endometrium is involved, it is considered endometrial cancer with cervical extension (FIGO).
- Pattern of metastases similar to that of epidermoid carcinoma of cervix, but local extension and node metastases appear earlier.
- Treatment similar to that of epidermoid carcinoma of cervix.
- Overall 5-year survival lower than for epidermoid carcinoma of cervix (stage I, 75%; II, 50%).

c. *Endometrioid adenocarcinoma of cervix*

- Constitutes 20% of adenocarcinomas of cervix.
- Difficult to distinguish from cervical extension of endometrial adenocarcinoma.
- Associated with foci of squamous metaplasia.

d. *Clear cell adenocarcinoma* (mesonephroid type adenocarcinoma)
   - Majority of tumors occur in patients whose mothers received DES during pregnancy (incidence 0.14–1.4/1000).
   - Some arise from mesonephric vestiges in the cervix and vaginal vault.
   - Gross: exophytic.
   - Microscopic: clear cells and hobnail cells with intraglandular papillary pattern in glands, tubules, or solid nests.

3. **Adenoepidermoid and adenosquamous carcinoma *(mixed carcinoma)***
   - Mixture of malignant epidermoid and glandular elements.
   - Endocervical glands replaced by an anaplastic epidermoid epithelium without alterations of the surface epithelium.
   - Adenoid pattern is maintained in most cases.
   - Often found in pregnancy, rarely discovered in its early stage, responsible for many barrel lesions.
   - Malignancy potential probably equal to that of the epidermoid variety stage for stage.
   - *Adenosquamous carcinoma:* maturation of metaplastic epidermoid elements; rare lesion.
   - *Glassy cell carcinoma* (Glucksmann and Cherry 1956).
   - Represents an undifferentiated form of adenoepidermoid carcinoma.
   - Rare (1.2% of all carcinomas of cervix).
   - Consists of invasive sheets of nests of malignant epithelial cells lying in a scant stroma.
     - Cells are large, polygonal or oval, and have distinct cell walls, ground glass or finely granular cytoplasm; prominent nuclei with

finely dispersed chromatin and prominent nucleoli; mitotic figures are numerous.
- Stroma consists of thin fibrous septa with prominent inflammatory cell infiltrate (eosinophils, lymphocytes, plasma cells).

- Early node metastases.
- Poor response to surgery or radiotherapy.

## D. Other primary malignancies

### 1. Sarcomas

a. *Leiomyosarcoma:* rare, diagnosis as for leiomyosarcoma of the uterus, based on mitotic figures per 10 HPF.

b. *Stromal sarcoma:* superficial lesion, treated with simple hysterectomy.

c. *Sarcoma botryoides:* pattern identical to lesion in vagina.

**2. Mixed mesodermal tumor:** like its counterpart in the fundus: atypical changes in epithelium and stroma, heterologous elements (cartilage, striated muscle cells).

### 3. Adenoid basal carcinoma

- Unusual lesion: patients in their sixties or seventies, occurs in the portio of the cervix, routinely associated with epidermoid CIS.
- Resembles the basal cell tumor of the skin: nests of small cells with dark regular nuclei in stroma.
- Locally invasive.
- Treatment: simple hysterectomy.

### 4. Adenoid cystic carcinoma

- Occurs mostly in elderly multigravid blacks.
- Like the tumor of the salivary gland.
- Locally aggressive and metastasizes late.
- Microscopic: nests or anastomosing cords of

uniform round or oval cells with scanty cytoplasm and hyperchromatic nuclei. Hyaline bodies within nests of cells.

- Treatment similar to that of invasive epidermoid carcinoma of the cervix.

## E. Metastatic tumors of cervix

1. **From endometrial adenocarcinoma, vaginal carcinoma, and ovarian carcinoma.**
2. **Choriocarcinoma.**
3. **Breast carcinoma.**
4. **Gastric carcinoma.**
5. **Leukemia.**

## Suggested Readings

1. Berek JS, Hacker NF, Fu YS, Sokale Jr, Leuchter RC, Lagasse LD. Adenocarcinoma of the uterine cervix: Histologic variables associated with lymph node metastasis and survival. *Obstet Gynecol* 65:46, 1985.
2. Creasman WT, Fetter BF, Clarke Pearson DL, Kaufman L, Parker RT. Management of stage IA carcinoma of the cervix. *Am J Obstet Gynecol* 153:164, 1985.
3. Crissman JD, Makuch R, Budhraja M. Histopathologic grading of squamous cell carcinoma of the uterine cervix: An evaluation of 70 Stage IB patients. *Cancer* 55:1590, 1985.
4. Dinh TV, Woodruff JD. Adenoid cystic and adenoid basal carcinomas of the cervix. *Obstet Gynecol* 65:705, 1985.
5. Fu YS, Reagan JW, Hsiu JG, Storaasli JP, Wentz WB. Adenocarcinoma and mixed carcinoma of the uterine cervix I: A clinicopathologic study. *Cancer* 49:2560, 1982.
6. Fu YS, Reagan JW, Richart RM. Precursors of cervical cancer. *Cancer Surv* 2:359, 1983.

7. Glucksmann A, Cherry CP. Incidence, histology and response to radiation of mixed carcinomas (adenoacanthomas) of the uterine cervix. *Cancer* 9:971, 1956.
8. Kaminski PF, Norris HJ. Minimal deviation carcinoma (adenoma malignum) of the cervix. *Int J Gynecol Pathol* 2:141, 1983.
9. Meisels A, Morin C, Casas-Cordero M. Human papilloma virus infection of the uterine cervix. *Int J Gynecol Pathol* 1:75, 1982.
10. Ostor AG, Pagano R, Davoren RAM, Fortune DW, Chanen W, Rome R. Adenocarcinoma in situ of the cervix. *Int J Gynecol Pathol* 3:179, 1984.
11. Richart RM. Cervical intraepithelial neoplasia. In: Sommers SC (ed). *Pathology Annual,* pp. 301–328. New York: Appleton-Century-Crofts, 1973.
12. Richart RM, Barron BA. A followup study of patients with cervical dysplasia. *Am J Obstet Gynecol* 105:386, 1969.
13. Yajima A, Fukuda M, Noda K. Histopathological findings concerning the morphogenesis of mixed carcinoma of the uterine cervix. *Gynecol Oncol* 18:157, 1984.

# 5. The Endometrium

I. Embryology
II. Normal histology
III. Physiologic changes
IV. Iatrogenic changes
V. Inflammations
VI. Benign tumors: endometrial polyps
VII. Hyperplasia
VIII. Carcinoma
IX. Tumors metastatic to the endometrium

## I. Embryology

- Corpus uteri arises from fusion of the caudal portions of the müllerian ducts (uterovaginal primordium).
- Lumen of ducts is lined by columnar epithelium from which the endometrial glands later proliferate.
- Endometrial glands induce formation of stroma and smooth muscle from the adjacent mesenchyme.
- Epithelium, stroma, and smooth muscle are of mesodermal origin.

## II. Normal histology

### A. Endometrial glands

- Epithelium composed of tall columnar cells with basal, elongated nuclei in the proliferative phase.
- Subnuclear vacuoles, evidence of ovulation.
- Cells with frayed and ragged appearance and with round, vesicular nuclei in the secretory phase.

### B. Surface epithelium

- Gradual increase in height from cuboidal to tall columnar at ovulation.
- Can have mucoid, or squamous metaplasia, or ciliated cell under the influence of estrogen.

### C. Stroma

- Cells with little cytoplasm and with large dark spindle or round nucleus.
- Become enlarged, polyhedral, and pale staining (pseudodecidua) in the secretory phase.
- *Note:* The endometrium is divided into two zones.
  1. **Functional:** consists of compact and spongy layers that are responsive to hormones.
  2. **Nonfunctional:** adjacent to myometrium consists of a basal layer from which the endometrium regenerates after each menstruation ("reserve cell layer" of the endometrium). This basal layer is not subject to the influence of progesterone.

## III. Physiologic changes

### A. Dating the endometrium

1. **Proliferative phase**
   a. Early proliferative (4th to 7th day)
      - Thin regenerating surface epithelium.
      - Straight tubular (non-coiled) short glands with mitoses.
      - Compact spindled stroma with some mitotic activity.

   b. Mid proliferative (8th to 10th day)
      - Columnar surface epithelium.
      - Loosely coiled and elongated glands with

pseudostratified nuclei, abundant mitoses in the epithelium.
- Stromal edema with mitoses.

c. Late proliferative (11th to 14th day)
- Undulant columnar surface epithelium.
- Tortuous (tightly coiled) glands with mitoses and pseudostratification
- Dense, actively growing stroma.

**2. Secretory phase**

- No microscopic changes apparent till 36–48 hours after ovulation. Following are histologic changes which permit dating of the endometrium, beginning postovulatory day 2 (POD 2).
    - *POD 2:* subnuclear vacuoles in gland epithelium.
    - *POD 3:* orderly row of nuclei with large vacuoles below.
    - *POD 4:* vacuoles above and below nuclei.
    - *POD 6:* peak of intraluminal secretion.
    - *POD 8:* peak of stromal edema.
    - *POD 9:* prominent spiral arterioles.
    - *POD 10:* thick periarterial cuffs of predecidua.
    - *POD 11:* predecidua under the surface epithelium, mitoses in stroma.
    - *POD 12:* solid sheets of predecidua. Infiltration of stromal granulocytes.
    - *POD 13:* marked infiltration of stromal granulocytes.
    - *POD 14:* focal necrosis and hemorrhage in stroma.
    - Menses: crumbling stroma, glandular breakup, and hemorrhage.

- Dating should be based on the most advanced area expressed as a 48-hour interval (e.g., POD 9–10). Subnuclear vacuolation should be present in at least 50% of the functional glands to confirm ovulation.
- Luteal phase defect: occurs in 3–5% of infertile population. Normal secretory appearance, but histology dating lags more than 2 days behind menstrual dating (in relation to the onset of the subsequent menstrual period). Treatment with progesterone vaginal suppositories, clomiphene citrate, or human menopausal gonadotropin.

### B. Pregnancy

- Glands are hypersecretory and show Arias Stella reaction, which consists of tufting and budding of glandular epithelium, large cells with clear or vacuolated cytoplasm and slight nuclear atypia (enlargement, hyperchromatism, nucleoli, sometimes mitosis). May be confused with clear cell adenocarcinoma.
- Stromal cells become decidual cells: large and polygonal, wide zone of cytoplasm surrounding the nucleus, arranged in mosaic fashion.

### C. Menopause

- Surface epithelium thin, low cuboidal.
- Gland epithelium low cuboidal, inactive. Glands sparse, at times cystic.
- Stroma fibrotic.

## IV. Iatrogenic changes

### A. IUD *(intrauterine devices)*

- Focal or extensive chronic inflammation, focal squamous metaplasia of surface epithelium.

- Actinomycosis (Actinomyces israelii, gram-positive anaerobic organism).
- *Unilateral* tubo-ovarian abscess may occur subsequent to an endometritis.
- IUD with progesterone: decidual reaction and atrophy of glands in superficial endometrium.

### B. OCA *(oral contraceptive agents)*

- Glands straight, inactive with no mitoses or secretion.
- Stroma with pseudodecidual changes, prominent venules, sparse scattering of lymphocytes, and polymorphonuclear leukocytes (stromal glandular disparity).

**C. Progestins:** decidual reaction and glandular suppression.

**D. Clomiphene:** like normal menstrual cycle.

## V. Inflammations

### A. Acute endometritis

- Etiology: puerperal infections (anaerobic Streptococci, Escherichia coli, Bacteroides, Pseudomonas, and rarely Clostridium perfringens), gonorrhea, actinomycosis (IUD), Chlamydia trachomatis.
- Gross: congestion, edema, swelling of endometrium in mild forms, purulent surface with ulceration in virulent forms, infiltration of myometrium, and parametrium and thrombophlebitis of uterine and pelvic vessels.
- Microscopic: diffuse infiltration of the stroma by polymorphonuclear leukocytes; collections of leukocytes in lumen of glands, vascular congestion, and stromal edema.
- Treatment: antibiotics.

### B. Chronic endometritis

- Etiology: IUD, retained gestational tissue (hyalinized decidua, ghost villi), tuberculosis, submucous myoma.
- Gross: pale and swollen endometrium.
- Microscopic: chronic inflammation; round cell and plasma cell infiltration (lymphocytes and lymphoid follicles are *normally* present in endometrium); stromal edema and vascular congestion.
- Treatment: according to etiology.

### C. Tuberculous endometritis

- Secondary to tuberculosis of the tube.
- Microscopic: tubercles with epithelioid and giant cells, sometimes caseation.

### D. Postmenopausal endometritis

- Develops in postmenopausal women, may cause bleeding.
- Microscopic: thin inactive endometrium, blood vessels thick-walled and calcified, stromal infiltration by lymphocytes and plasma cells, focal squamous metaplasia of surface epithelium (ichthyosis uteri, if extensive).

## VI. **Benign tumors:** endometrial polyps

- Consist of projections of endometrium into the uterine cavity.
- Clinical: most are asymptomatic, bleeding with large, ulcerated, or pedunculated polyps that protrude into cervix or vagina.
- Microscopic: epithelium on three sides, core of fibrous stroma with thick-walled vessels. Three types of endometrial polyps.

  - *Polyps with functional endometrium:* normal pattern is like that of the surrounding endometrium.
  - *Polyps with immature endometrium:* hyperplastic pattern (Swiss cheese type adenomatous hyperplasia), atrophic pattern (low columnar to cuboidal glandular epithelium frequent in postmenopausal women).
  - *Adenomyomatous polyp:* endometrial elements and involuntary muscle tissue.
- Malignant degeneration low (0.45–3.7%); (essential to study the polyp base for differential diagnosis between malignant degeneration of a polyp and polypoid adenocarcinoma).
- Fifteen percent of endometrial malignancies in postmenopausal women are associated with benign polyps (Peterson and Novak); essential to perform a complete curettage when finding is a benign endometrial polyp in a woman with postmenopausal bleeding.

## VII. Hyperplasia

**A. Definition:** proliferation of glands and of stroma, result of prolonged and persistent estrogenic stimulation of endometrium.

**B. Gross:** endometrium thick, velvety, creamy yellow, sometimes polypoid, measuring more than 5 mm in thickness.

**C. Types of hyperplasia:** cystic hyperplasia, adenomatous hyperplasia, atypical hyperplasia.

1. **Cystic hyperplasia *(swiss cheese hyperplasia)***
   - Glands large and cystically dilated.
   - Cells in glands are elongated, pseudostratified, and with nuclei perpendicular to basement membrane.
   - Mitotic figures present but not numerous.

- Squamous and tubal metaplasia common.
- Stroma with plump spindled cells.
- Different from cystic changes of atrophic endometria in postmenopausal women in whom the epithelium is inactive and the stroma is fibrotic.
- Incidence of subsequent malignancy low (1–5%).

2. **Adenomatous hyperplasia**
   - Increase in number of glands that exhibit budding and branching.
   - Cells in glands that are elongated or round, stratified or pseudostratified.
   - Stroma cellular, sometimes edematous, and diminished in amount.
   - Incidence of subsequent malignancy: 10–25%.

3. **Atypical hyperplasia**
   - Glands crowded with budding and branching.
   - Stroma scarce (ratio of glands to stroma greater than 1).
   - Most important: atypia in glandular epithelium characterized by loss of cellular orientation, prominent stratification, eosinophilic cytoplasm, round nuclei, with chromatin clearing or clumping and prominent nucleoli. Atypical mitoses may be numerous.
   - Atypia may be

   a. *Mild:* glands minimally crowded; few papillary infoldings; cells radially oriented with only focal loss of polarity; minimal atypia of cells.

   b. *Severe:* glands closely packed and with minimal stroma; complex glandular infoldings leading to cribriform pattern (glands back to back); complete loss of cell polarity; cells are atypical; difficult to distinguish from adenocarcinoma.

c. *Moderate:* histologic feature between mild and severe.

- Incidence of subsequent malignancy high (25–50%).
- The International Society of Gynecological Pathologists has proposed a new classification of endometrial hyperplasia: simple hyperplasia, complex hyperplasia (adenomatous without atypia), and atypical hyperplasia (adenomatous with atypia).
- Mean duration of progression of hyperplasia without atypia and atypical hyperplasia to carcinoma is respectively 10 and 4 years.

## D. Metaplasia of glandular epithelium in hyperplasia

1. **Tubal metaplasia *(ciliated cell metaplasia).***
2. **Eosinophilic metaplasia:** enlarged glandular cells with eosinophilic cytoplasm, bland nuclei.
3. **Mucinous metaplasia.**
4. **Squamous metaplasia *(or adenoacanthosis):*** frequent; prognosis depends on glandular component. (Morules: spheric or ellipsoid aggregate of cytologically bland squamous cells, can be confused with adenocarcinoma.)

## E. Foam cells

- Associated with endometrial hyperplasias and 15% adenocarcinomas; are altered endometrial stromal cells.
- Consist of large polygonal cells with small central nuclei, finely vacuolated cytoplasm, and sharply defined borders.
- No clinical significance.

**F. Treatment:** depends on the age of the patient and the type of hyperplasia. Treat with surgery (hysterectomy) or progestins.

# VIII. Carcinoma

- Average age: 57 years.
- Most frequent complaint: abnormal uterine bleeding (mostly menopausal).
- Clinical association with endometrial adenocarcinoma: late menopause, obesity, hypertension, low parity, diabetes, increased incidence of breast carcinoma.

## A. FIGO staging

- *Stage I:* Carcinoma is confined to the corpus.
    - *IA:* tumor limited to endometrium.
    - *IB:* invasion to less than half of myometrium.
    - *IC:* invasion to more than half of myometrium.
- *Stage II:* Carcinoma has involved the corpus and cervix.
    - *IIA:* endocervical glandular involvement only.
    - *IIB:* cervical stromal invasion.
- *Stage III:* Carcinoma has extended outside the uterus.
    - *IIIA:* tumor invasion of serosa and/or adnexae and/or positive peritoneal cytology.
    - *IIIB:* vaginal metastases.
    - *IIIC:* metastases to pelvic and/or para-aortic lymph nodes.
- *Stage IV:* Carcinoma has extended outside the true pelvis or has involved the mucosa of the bladder or rectum.
    - *IVA:* tumor invasion of bladder and/or bowel mucosa.
    - *IVB:* distant metastases including intraabdominal and/or inguinal lymph node.

## B. FIGO grading: degree of differentiation

- *G1:* 5% or less of a nonsquamous or nonmorular solid growth pattern.
- *G2:* 6–50% of a nonsquamous or nonmorular solid growth pattern.
- *G3:* more than 50% of a nonsquamous or nonmorular solid growth pattern.

## C. Gross

1. **Diffuse form:** endometrium thickened, irregularly polypoid with surface ulceration or necrosis. Can extend to the cervix (differs from polypoid hyperplasia which does not invade cervix), myometrium, and peritoneum.
2. **Circumscribed:** localized polypoid mass that may be totally removed during curettage.

## D. Microscopic

- Glands increased in number, crowding (back to back) with intraglandular bridging and no intervening stroma.
- Random piling of cells into sheets or masses.
- Atypical cells with eosinophilic cytoplasm, nuclear abnormalities (hyperchromatism, pleomorphism, chromatin clearing or clumping, prominent nucleoli), mitotic figures (sometimes abnormal).
- Karyorrhectic debris and acute inflammatory cells within the glandular lumina.
- Morphologic parameters important to prognosis: grade of tumor, depth of invasion of myometrium, and positive peritoneal cytology.

## E. Clinical

- Treatment: total abdominal hysterectomy with bilateral salpingo-oophorectomy (TAH-BSO) and selective pelvic lymphadenectomy followed by whole pelvic irradiation depending on the extent of myometrial invasion (more than half) or grade (grade 3).

- Lymph node metastasis in stage I: grade 1, 2%; grade 2, 11%; grade 3, 27%.
- Five-year survival
  - Stage I, 74%; stage II, 57%; stage III, 29%; stage IV, 9% (Kottmeier).
  - Grade 1, 81%; grade 2, 74%; grade 3, 50% (Jones).
- Treatment of recurrences: hormonotherapy (progestins) and chemotherapy (doxorubicin [Adriamycin], cisplatin, etc.). Response poor.

## F. Histopathologic classification of carcinomas of the endometrium

1. **Endometrioid (or typical endometrial) adenocarcinoma:** as above. Variants: papillary carcinoma, secretory carcinoma, ciliated carcinoma.

   a. *Papillary carcinoma:* thin, delicate papillary fronds covered by stratified columnar epithelial cells with atypical nuclei. Excellent prognosis.

   b. *Secretory carcinoma:* cells with subnuclear or supranuclear vacuoles that resemble early secretory endometrium. Good prognosis.

   c. *Ciliated carcinoma:* rare, associated with exogenous estrogen treatment. Good prognosis.

2. **Adenoacanthoma *(adenocarcinoma with squamous differentiation)***
   - Gross: frequently exophytic lesions.
   - Squamous metaplasia (benign) in adenocarcinoma.

- Prognosis depends on the differentiation of the glandular element (often well differentiated).

3. **Clear cell adenocarcinoma**
   - Derived from müllerian epithelium.
   - Patterns: papillary, glandular, sheets, or tubules with clear cells and hobnail cells, psammoma bodies (in 15% of papillary clear cell adenocarcinoma).
   - Slightly worse prognosis than the usual adenocarcinoma (5-year survival, stage I, 44%).
4. **Papillary serous carcinoma:**
   - Different from papillary endometrioid carcinoma.
   - Histologically identical to serous carcinoma of ovary: papillary fronds consisting of delicate fibrovascular cores, covered by stratified and marked atypical cells (nuclear pleomorphism, hyperchromasia, macronucleoli, mitoses). Psammoma bodies may be present in ⅓ of cases.
   - Extensive invasion of myometrium with permeation of lymphatics and vascular channels and frequent dissemination beyond uterus.
   - Very poor prognosis.
   - Patients should receive adjuvant chemotherapy or irradiation.
5. **Mixed adenosquamous carcinoma**
   - Malignant squamous elements mixed with malignant glandular elements.
   - Early invasion of myometrium.
   - Prognosis poor: 30–40% 5-year survival.
6. **Epidermoid carcinoma**
   - Extremely rare lesion (21 cases recorded).
   - Arises from patches of squamous metaplasia in the columnar epithelium (ichthyosis uteri).

• Depth of invasion is the most significant prognostic factor.

## IX. Tumors metastatic to the endometrium

• Carcinoma of cervix.
• Endometrioid carcinoma of ovaries can coexist with adenocarcinoma of endometrium as 2 primary tumors (⅓ of cases—Scully). Multifocal disease, good prognosis (Woodruff).
• Breast carcinoma, gastric carcinoma, melanoma.
• Adenocarcinoma of colon, pancreas, and kidney.

### Suggested Readings

1. Arias-Stella JA. Atypical endometrial changes produced by chorionic tissue. *Hum Pathol* 3:450, 1972.
2. Boronow RC, Morrow CP, Creasman WT, et al. Surgical staging in endometrial cancer: Clinical-pathologic findings of a prospective study. *Obstet Gynecol* 53:825, 1984.
3. Chen J, Trost DC, Wilkinson EJ. Endometrial papillary adenocarcinomas: Two clinicopathologic types. *Int J Gynecol Pathol* 4:279, 1985.
4. Connelly PJ, Alberhasky RC, Christopherson WM. Carcinoma of the endometrium III: Analysis of 865 cases of adenocarcinoma and adenoacanthoma. *Obstet Gynecol* 59:569, 1982.
5. DiSaia PJ, Creasman WT, Boronow MD, Blessing JA. Risk factors and recurrent patterns in Stage I endometrial cancer. *Am J Obstet Gynecol* 151:1009, 1985.
6. Hendrickson MR, Kempson RL. Endometrial epithelial metaplasias proliferations frequently misdiagnosed as adenocarcinoma: Report of 89 cases and proposed classification. *Am J Surg Pathol* 4:525, 1980.
7. Hendrickson M, Ross J, Eifel P, Martinez A, Kempson R. Uterine papillary serous carcinoma: A highly

malignant form of endometrial adenocarcinoma. *Am J Surg Pathol* 6:93, 1982.

8. Jones GS. Luteal phase defects. In: Behrman SJ, Kistner RW (eds). *Progress in Infertility,* 2d ed., pp. 299–324. Boston: Little Brown, 1975.
9. Kurman RJ, Kaminski PF, Norris HJ. The behavior of endometrial hyperplasia: A long-term study of "untreated" hyperplasia in 170 patients. *Cancer* 56:403, 1985.
10. Kurman RJ, Norris HJ. Evaluation of criteria for distinguishing atypical endometrial hyperplasia from well-differentiated carcinoma. *Cancer* 49:2547, 1982.
11. Norris HJ, Tavassoli FA, Kurman RJ. Endometrial hyperplasia and carcinoma: Diagnostic considerations. *Am J Surg Pathol* 7:839, 1983.
12. Noyes RW, Hertig AT, Rock J. Dating the endometrial biopsy. *Fertil Steril* 1:3, 1950.
13. Peterson WF, Novak ER. Endometrial polyps. *Obstet Gynecol* 8:40, 1956.
14. Wentz AC, Herbert CM, Maxson WS, Garner CH. Outcome of progesterone treatment of luteal phase inadequacy. *Fertil Steril* 41:856, 1984.

# 6. The Myometrium

I. Embryology
II. Histology
III. Benign tumors
IV. Malignant tumors

## I. Embryology: see Endometrium (Chapter 5).

## II. Histology

- Broad interlacing bundles of spindled smooth muscle cells with blunt-end fusiform nuclei.
- Islands of dense connective tissue with many arteries and veins, between the muscle bundles.
- Hyperplasia and hypertrophy of myometrial cells during pregnancy (from 20 μm to 600 μm long).

## III. Benign tumors

### A. Adenomyosis

- Not a true tumor.
- Characterized by a benign invasion of the uterine musculature by the endometrium.
- Found in 25–40% of all hysterectomy specimens.

- Gross: uterus enlarged, posterior wall often thicker than anterior wall. Cut surface presents a diffuse, symmetric thickness of the muscular wall with whorled, trabeculated appearance and areas of dark, chocolate-colored blood.
- Microscopic: endometrial tissue should be at least one high power field ($10 \times 40$) below the basal endometrium. Aberrant endometrium can be nonfunctioning or functioning (secretory, pregnancy changes).
- Clinical: menorrhagia, dysmenorrhea.
- Malignant change infrequent. Prognosis excellent with adenocarcinoma in adenomyosis (not invasive cancer).
- Treatment: cyclic hormones or prostaglandin synthetase inhibitors. Hysterectomy is definitive treatment.

## B. Leiomyoma *(fibroid)*

- Most common pelvic tumor: 20% of women over 30 years old harbor uterine myomas.
- Location: submucous, interstitial, and subserous (can be intraligamentary or parasitic).
- Gross: firm whitish nodule, cut surface has a whorled trabeculation. Pseudocapsule of areolar tissue permits myomectomy.
- Microscopic: uniform spindle muscle cells, with uniform rod-like nuclei arranged in interlacing whorl pattern.
- Treatment: myomectomy or total hysterectomy.

### 1. Extrauterine leiomyomas

a. *Intravenous leiomyomatosis:* myomas arise in pelvic veins, then migrate to vena cava, heart, lungs. Microscopic appearance benign—clinical course benign and prolonged. Treatment: hysterectomy and, if possible, removal of the extrauterine lesion.

b. *Leiomyomatosis peritonealis disseminata (LPD)*
   - Rare (15 cases recorded), chiefly in pregnant patients.
   - Gross: numerous small myomas in omentum, peritoneal cavity, small and large bowels, bladder; simulate carcinomatosis.
   - Microscopic: benign myomas.
   - Treatment: TAH-BSO in some cases; some regress after pregnancy.

**2. Secondary changes in myomas**

a. *Hyaline:* most common.

b. *Cystic degeneration.*

c. *Calcareous degeneration.*

d. *Infection and suppuration (submucous myomas).*

e. *Necrosis (pedunculated myomas), carneous degeneration in pregnancy.*

f. *Sarcomatous change:* rare (0.5%).

**3. Other histologic types of leiomyomas**

a. *Cellular leiomyoma:* soft, rubbery, gray, composed of closely spaced elongated cells with uniform, bland nuclei. Benign.

b. *Bizarre leiomyoma (atypical leiomyoma):* occurs in ischemic myomas during pregnancy and in women taking OCA. Consists of muscle cells with pleomorphic, enlarged hyperchromatic nuclei and giant cell formation, but no mitoses or less than 2 mitotic figures per high power field (2 MF/HPF); can be mistaken for leiomyosarcoma. Benign.

c. *Epithelioid leiomyoma (leiomyoblastoma):* cells are rounded or polygonal and have clear or eosinophilic cytoplasm arranged in cords or nests. Benign if less than 5 MF/10 HPF (Kurman and Norris).

### C. Adenomatoid tumor *(mesothelioma)*

- Rare, resembles leiomyoma, grayish white, 0.5–2 cm in diameter.
- Considered a benign mesothelioma (similar to tubal lesion).
- Microscopic: gland-like spaces lined by flat or cuboidal cells and surrounded by a dense stroma or smooth muscle.
- Treatment: excision of lesion or hysterectomy.

### D. Stromal nodule

- Almost always solitary; can vary in size from microscopic to more than 6 cm in diameter.
- Consists of a spheric aggregate of bland endometrial stromal cells in the myometrium.
- Pushing margins; no lymphatic or vascular invasion.
- Mitotic figures less than 10 per 10 HPF (Norris and Taylor).
- Clinical features: abnormal uterine bleeding with large lesions.
- Benign, treated with total abdominal hysterectomy (TAH).
- Prognosis excellent.

### E. Stromatosis *(endolymphatic stromal myosis)*

- Gross: tumor within myometrium or protruding into endometrial cavity as polypoid mass.
- Microscopic: infiltrating margins; nuclei usually bland, less than 10 MF/10 HPF; vascular and lymphatic involvement common (Taylor and Norris).

- May extend outside the uterus and can metastasize.
- Pelvic recurrences common (50%) unless tumor small.
- Considered a *low grade stromal sarcoma.*
- Clinical: abnormal uterine bleeding, pelvic or abdominal pain, enlarged uterus.
- Treatment: TAH; progestogens without interruption, for recurrence, or if stroma has penetrated more than 50% of the myometrium (Woodruff).
- Prognosis: relatively favorable, even with repeated local recurrences.

## IV. Malignant tumors

### A. Ober classification of sarcomas

#### 1. Pure sarcomas

a. *Homologous*
   i. Stromal sarcoma (derived from endometrial stroma).
   ii. Leiomyosarcoma (derived from myoma or normal myometrium).
   iii. Angiosarcoma.
   iv. Fibrosarcoma.

b. *Heterologous* (extremely rare)
   i. Rhabdomyosarcoma.
   ii. Chondrosarcoma.
   iii. Osteosarcoma.
   iv. Liposarcoma.

#### 2. Mixed pure sarcomas *(homologous or heterologous)*

#### 3. Mixed mesodermal (müllerian) tumors

a. *Homologous:* carcinosarcoma.

b. *Heterologous:* mixed mesodermal tumors (mixed müllerian tumor).

## B. GOG classification of sarcomas

### 1. Leiomyosarcoma

- Average age: 52 years, 20% nulliparous.
- Clinical: menometrorrhagia or postmenopausal bleeding, pelvic pain, abdominal mass.
- Incidence of sarcomatous degeneration in a myoma: 0.5% or less.
- Gross: soft myoma, necrotic, "raw pork" appearance; diffuse enlargement of the uterine wall in primary leiomyosarcoma.
- Microscopic: differential diagnosis to exclude cellular myoma and bizarre myoma. Diagnosis chiefly based on number of mitotic figures per HPF in the most active area (Novak and Woodruff).

| | |
|---|---|
| 1–4 MF/HPF | 100% 5-year survival |
| 2–5 MF/HPF | 77% 5-year survival |
| 6–10 MF/HPF | 38% 5-year survival |
| > 10 MF/HPF | 0% 5-year survival |

- Other authors consider number of MF/10 HPF (counting at least 40 HPF).

| | |
|---|---|
| < 5 MF/10 HPF | Benign |
| 5–9 MF/10 HPF | Uncertain potential for malignancy |
| > 10 MF/10 HPF | Malignant |

- Five-year survival (Dinh and Woodruff)

| | |
|---|---|
| 1–4 MF/10 HPF | 94.6% |
| 5–9 MF/10 HPF | 48.2% |
| > 10 MF/10 HPF | 24.2% |

- Features for good prognostic include: premenopausal status, few MF/HPF, absence of necrosis, presence of hyaline degeneration, localization in a myoma, early stage.
- Treatment: TAH-BSO. Adjuvant chemotherapy (Adriamycin) of no value.

- Five-year survival: stage I, 56%; stages II–IV, 7% (Salazar 1978).

2. **Stromal sarcoma.**
   - Represents the malignant end of stromal proliferation (stromal nodule—stromatosis—stromal sarcoma).
   - Rarest of the sarcomas.
   - Clinical: menometrorrhagia, postmenopausal bleeding, abdominal mass, pelvic pain.
   - Gross: white or grayish pink, soft and fleshy polypoid excrescence in endometrial cavity.
   - Microscopic: sheets of stromal cells with mitoses more than 10 MF/ 10 HPF, nuclear atypia common, vascular and lymphatic invasion.
   - Spread of tumor is lymphatic and hematogenous.
   - Treatment: TAH-BSO, possibly progestogens or adjuvant chemotherapy.
   - Prognosis poor: 5-year survival, stage I, 55%; stages II–IV, 12% (Salazar).
   - Features for poor prognosis: size of tumor (greater than 4 cm) and extrauterine extension.

3. **Malignant mixed mesodermal *(müllerian)* tumors**
   - Represent 3–6% of all uterine cancers.
   - Occur in older patients (average age 62), aggressive tumor.
   - Ten to thirty percent had irradiation to the pelvis (11–16 years previously).
   - Clinical: postmenopausal bleeding, vaginal discharge, pelvic pain, abdominal mass.
   - Gross: soft and polypoid tumor in endometrial cavity, sometimes protruding through

cervix (⅓ of cases), sometimes large and bulky.

- Microscopic: admixture of carcinomatous and sarcomatous elements.
- Clinical: postmenopausal bleeding, vaginal discharge, pelvic pain, abdominal mass.

a. *Carcinoma (glandular or squamous) with stromal sarcoma or leiomyo-sarcoma:* homologous mixed mesodermal tumor, or carcinosarcoma.

b. Carcinoma with chondrosarcoma or rhabdomyosarcoma or osteosarcoma: heterologous mixed mesodermal tumor.

- Myometrial invasion frequent at the time of diagnosis (60%—DiSaia).
- Early lymph node metastasis (35% in stage I–DiSaia).
- Treatment: TAH-BSO. Radiation therapy to the pelvis may provide local pelvic control. Adjuvant chemotherapy has little effect.
- Factors determining prognosis: depth of myometrial invasion and extension of tumor (lymphatic and hematogenous spread). No difference in survival between homologous and heterologous tumors.
- Prognosis poor: 5-year survival, stage I, 50%; stages II–IV, 12% (Salazar).
- Metastases resemble adenocarcinoma in 75–80% of cases.

**4. Other uterine sarcomas**

a. *Adenosarcoma (müllerian adenosarcoma)*

- Occurs at all ages.
- Gross: resembles polypoid growth.
- Microscopic: epithelium resembles proliferative or inactive endometrium, stroma atypical, with mitoses (> 4 MF/10 HPF).

- Treatment: TAH-BSO followed by irradiation of entire pelvis (Morrow and Townsend).
- One-third recur from 6 months to 10 years.

b. *Lymphangiosarcoma, rhabdomyosarcoma, and liposarcoma:* rare.

## Suggested Readings


1. Dinh TV, Woodruff JD. Leiomyosarcoma of the uterus. *Am J Obstet Gynecol* 144:817, 1982.
2. George M, Pejovic MH, Kramer A, Gynecologic Cooperating Group of French Oncology Centers. Uterine sarcomas; prognostic factors and treatment modalities: Study on 209 patients. *Gynecol Oncol* 24:58, 1986.
3. Hannigan EV, Freedman RS, Rutledge FN. Adjuvant chemotherapy in early uterine sarcoma. *Gynecol Oncol* 15:56, 1983.
4. Kahanpaa KV, Wahlstrom T, Grohn P, Heinonen E, Nieminen U, Widholm O. Sarcomas of the uterus: A clinicopathologic study of 119 patients. *Obstet Gynecol* 67:417, 1986.
5. Kempson RL, Bari W. Uterine sarcomas: Classification, diagnosis and prognosis. *Human Pathol* 1:331, 1970.
6. Kurman RJ, Norris HJ. Mesenchymal tumors of the uterus VI: Epithelioid smooth muscle tumors including leiomyoblastoma and clear cell leiomyoma; a clinical and pathologic analysis of 26 cases. *Cancer* 37:1853, 1976.
7. Marchese MJ, Liskow AS, Crum CP, McCaffrey RM, et al. Uterine sarcomas: A clinicopathologic study, 1965–1981. *Gynecol Oncol* 18:299, 1984.
8. Norris HJ, Parmley T. Mesenchymal tumors of the uterus V: Intravenous leiomyomatosis; a clinical and pathologic study of 14 cases. *Cancer* 36:2164, 1975.
9. Ober WB. Uterine sarcomas: Histogenesis and taxonomy. *Ann N.Y. Acad Sci* 75:568, 1959.

10. Spanos WJ Jr, Wharton JT, Gomez L, Fletcher GH, et al. Malignant mixed müllerian tumors of the uterus. *Cancer* 53:311, 1984.

11. Thatcher SS, Woodruff JD. Uterine stromatosis: A report of 33 cases. *Obstet Gynecol* 59:428, 1982.

12. Wheelock JB, Krebs HB, Schneider V, Goplerud DR. Uterine sarcoma: Analysis of prognostic variables in 71 cases. *Am J Obstet Gynecol* 151:1016, 1985.

# 7. The Fallopian Tubes

I. Embryology
II. Anatomy and histology
III. Physiologic changes
IV. Inflammations
V. Other conditions
VI. Benign tumors
VII. Malignancies

## I. Embryology:

fallopian tubes develop from the cranial unfused portions of the müllerian ducts.

## II. Anatomy and histology

- Anatomy: interstitial (1 cm), isthmic (2 cm), ampullary (6 cm), and fimbriated (infundibulum) (1 cm) portions.
- Histology: three coats—serous, muscular (outer longitudinal, middle circular, inner longitudinal), and mucosal (with lamina propria between epithelium and muscularis).
- Mucosa disposed in longitudinal folds; three or four at the inner end of the tube and many folds at the fimbriated end.
- Epithelium composed of four types of cells: ciliated, secretory, intercalary (or peg cells), indifferent.

### A. Ciliated cells

- Pale cytoplasm with clear halo around nucleus.
- Nucleus round or ovoid, situated near the ciliated end, pale on hematoxylin and eosin (H & E) stain.
- Height changes during cycle: lower in postmenstrual phase and pregnancy.
- Presence of about 50 cilia per cell.

### B. Secretory cells

- Cytoplasm dark and uniform.
- Nucleus dark; in the secretory phase, projects into the lumen, like dome.
- Height varies during cycle: lower during menstruation and pregnancy.

### C. Intercalary cells *(or peg cells)*

- Abundant during premenstrual and menstrual periods.
- Long, slender rod-like nuclei and small amount of cytoplasm, squeezed by adjoining cells.
- Represent secretory cells in transitional stages.

### D. Indifferent cells *(wandering cells)*

- Lie at the base of normal epithelium.
- May be the progenitor of epithelial and stromal elements (Woodruff and Pauerstein).
- Most are actually lymphocytes by electron microscopy.

## III. Physiologic changes

### A. Pregnancy

- Decrease in height of ciliated and secretory cells.
- Increase in number of peg cells.
- Arias-Stella pattern may be seen.

- Decidual reaction in lamina propria.
- Marked infiltration of lamina propria with polymorphonuclear cells in the postpartum (10%).

**B. Prepuberty:** epithelium low with both chief types of cells.

**C. Postmenopause:** epithelium low, although it may remain high for many years.

## IV. Inflammations

### A. Acute and subacute salpingitis

- Gross: tube red, swollen, turgid, with purulent discharge exuding from fimbriae. Tubes are affected nearly bilaterally, except in some patients with IUD (unilateral pelvic inflammatory disease [PID]).
- Microscopic
  - Mucosal rugae edematous.
  - Lamina propria infiltrated by polymorphonuclear leukocytes.
  - Marked engorgement of vessels.
  - Lumen filled with purulent exudate.
  - Can progress to pelvic abscess or tubo-ovarian abscess.
- Etiology: gonococcus (25–80%), Chlamydia trachomatis, Bacteroides, Peptococcus, Peptostreptococcus, E. coli.
- Treatment: antibiotics.

### B. Chronic salpingitis

#### 1. Pyosalpinx

- Sequel of gonorrheal salpingitis or other inflammatory process.
- Results from blockage of the tube and fim-

briae at different points, which causes tubal distention and retained purulent exudate.

- Gross: markedly distended tube with purulent exudate, often adherent to adjacent structures.
- Microscopic: distorted mucosal folds with flattened cells, stroma infiltrated with chronic inflammatory cells, mesothelium often reactive with adenomatous or papillary formations, psammoma bodies, giant cells, and bizarre patterns mimicking malignancy.
- Treatment: antibiotics and surgery.

**2. Hydrosalpinx**

- End result of pyosalpinx characterized by resorption of purulent exudate.
- Walls thin and translucent with clear watery fluid.

a. *Hydrosalpinx simplex:* One single lumen in the distended tube with flattened epithelium.

b. *Hydrosalpinx follicularis:* Many compartments in the distended tube from adherence of adjoining rugae.

- No treatment unless symptomatic.

## C. Salpingitis isthmica nodosa

- Probably results from the residue of a chronic interstitial salpingitis.
- Etiology still debatable: inflammation or adenomyosis-like origin.
- Gross: one or multiple firm nodules up to 2 cm at the isthmic portion of the tube.
- Microscopic: thickening of muscularis, numerous small tubal lumens throughout the muscularis. Minimal inflammatory infiltrate.
- High incidence of infertility and strong association with ectopic pregnancy.
- No treatment.

### D. Granulomatous salpingitis

#### 1. Tuberculous salpingitis

- Rare.
- Secondary to a focus elsewhere but almost always primary in the female genital tract: the bacilli reach the tube from the lungs, urinary tract, or abdominal cavity.
- Gross: similar to chronic salpingitis. Cross-section can show cheesy necrotic exudate and caseation of the tubal wall. Fimbriated end often everted and open (in contradistinction to its appearance in chronic salpingitis).
- Microscopic: granuloma with caseation and typical tubercles, striking adenomatous pattern of the mucosa which is mistaken for adenocarcinoma.
- Treatment: antituberculosis drugs and surgery.

#### 2. Actinomycosis

- Rare, associated with IUD.
- Microscopic: histiocytes, plasma cells, lymphocytes in abscess walls, and gram-positive filamentous clumps, sulfur granules.

#### 3. Lipogranulomatous salpingitis

- Caused by lipidol that is introduced during hysterosalpingogram.
- Microscopic: granulomata with epithelioid and giant cells.

## V. Other conditions of the fallopian tubes

### A. Tubal pregnancy

- Incidence 0.25–1% of all pregnancies.
- Ninety-six percent of ectopic pregnancies occur in the tube; 80% of all tubal pregnancies occur in the ampulla, 13% in the isthmus.

- Possible mechanisms: chronic salpingitis, tubal diverticula, increased tubal receptivity (endometriosis, decidual reaction), abnormal ovum, salpingitis isthmica nodosa.
- Pathology: trophoblast readily penetrates the mucosa and muscle; mucosa has limited ability to undergo decidualization; tubal lumen has limited ability to expand for growth of embryo. Ultimate outcome: perforation or rupture of the tube, or abortion through the infundibulum and death of the embryo.
- Gross: hematosalpinx with a site of perforation and hemoperitoneum.
- Microscopic: chorionic villi penetrating the muscularis, close to or through the serosa. Decidua often absent.
- Clinical: amenorrhea, pain, metrorrhagias; diagnosis by serum BHCG (beta subunit of human chorionic gonadotropin), ultrasound, culdocentesis; treatment with surgery (salpingostomy and salpingectomy).

### B. Prolapse of the tube

- Occurs as a rare complication of vaginal or abdominal hysterectomy.
- Clinical: vaginal discharge a few days to several years after hysterectomy, excrescence at the apex of vagina; biopsy shows tubal epithelium with inflammation.
- Treatment: salpingectomy.

## VI. Benign tumors

### A. Adenomatoid tumor *(mesothelioma)*

- Most common. Similar lesions found on uterine surface and in cul-de-sac.
- Gross: tumor 1–2 cm, near the cornua of fundus, yellow or whitish gray on section.

- Microscopic: small tubules lined by a flattened or low cuboidal epithelium.
- Treatment: excision.

### B. Endometriosis

- Seen in the interstitial portion of the tube.
- Microscopic: uterine glands and stroma.

### C. Papilloma, leiomyoma: rare.

### D. So-called "metaplastic tumor": probably an exaggerated Arias-Stella reaction.

## VII. Malignancies

### A. Primary carcinoma

- Rare, 0.2–0.5% of malignancies of the genital canal, seldom diagnosed preoperatively.
- Mean age: 52 years, affecting women of low parity.
- Clinical features: vaginal bleeding or profuse watery yellow or amber discharge, hydrops tubae profluens rare (colicky lower abdominal pain relieved by vaginal serosanguineous discharge).
- Staging: There is no FIGO staging classification for tubal carcinoma. The FIGO staging for ovarian cancer may be used.
  - *Stage O:* CIS limited to tubal mucosa.
  - *Stage I:* growth limited to fallopian tubes.
    - *IA:* one fallopian tube; no ascites; no tumor on external surface; tubal serosa intact.
    - *IB:* both fallopian tubes; no ascites; no tumor on external surface; tubal serosa intact.
    - *IC:* stage IA or IB but with tumor on the surface, tubal serosa ruptured, or with ascites containing malignant cells or with positive peritoneal cytology.

- *Stage II:* Tumor involving one or both tubes with pelvic extension.
  - *IIA:* extension or metastases to uterus and/or ovaries.
  - *IIB:* extension to other pelvic tissues.
  - *IIC:* IIA or IIB with ascites containing malignant cells or positive peritoneal washings.
- *Stage III:* tumor involving one or both fallopian tubes with peritoneal implants outside the pelvis and/or positive retroperitoneal or inguinal nodes; tumor limited to pelvis but with histologically proven malignant extension to small bowel or omentum.
  - *IIIA:* tumor limited to true pelvis with negative nodes but histologically confirmed microscopic seeding of the abdominal peritoneal surface.
  - *IIIB:* tumor of one or both fallopian tubes with histologically confirmed implants of abdominal peritoneal surfaces ($< 2$ cm in diameter), negative nodes.
  - *IIIC:* abdominal implants $> 2$ cm in diameter and/or positive retroperitoneal or inguinal nodes.
- *Stage IV:* growth involving one or both fallopian tubes with distant metastases (positive cytology in pleural effusion, parenchymal liver metastases, etc.).

- Gross: tube enlarged, sausage-shaped, and without adhesions to the surrounding structures. Neoplasm often arises in middle and outer third of the tube. Bilateral involvement in 15% of cases. Fimbriated end closed in half the cases.
- Microscopic: three types—papillary, papillary-alveolar, and alveolar-medullary (Hu, Taymor, and Hertig).
  - Dominant histologic variant: adenocarcinoma.
  - Histologic grade does not affect survival.

- *Papillary* (more common)
  - Papillae covered by a multilayered atypical epithelium.
  - Mitoses frequent.
  - Differential diagnosis to exclude tuberculosis.
- *Papillary-alveolar:* later stage of papillary with agglutination of papillary folds.
- *Alveolar-medullary:* Often tube and ovary are involved; tubal lesion is often considered secondary.

- Criteria for diagnosis of primary tubal cancer (Hu, Taymor, and Hertig)
  - Main tumor in the tube.
  - Microscopically, mucosa is chiefly involved and exhibits a papillary pattern.
  - If tubal wall is involved, transition between normal and malignant epithelium should be demonstrated.
- Bilateral in 20–40% of cases. Not metastatic. Demonstration of "tumor in paired organs" (Woodruff).
- Treatment: TAH-BSO, omentectomy with radiation or chemotherapy (doxorubicin, cisplatin, melphalan, progestins).
- Five-year survival: stage I, 72%; II, 38%; III, 18%; IV, 0% (Denham and Maclennan); all stages, 38% (Sedlis).

**B. Carcinoma in situ:** multilayered papillary epithelium with nuclear atypia and *mitoses*. Basement membrane intact. Prognosis good.

### C. Secondary or metastatic carcinoma

- More common than primary neoplasm; secondary to ovarian and fundal malignancies.
- Emboli of cancer cells in vascular channels of the adjacent mesosalpinx.

## D. Choriocarcinoma

- Rare as primary neoplasm (15 cases recorded).
- Secondary to extension from a primary in the uterus or ovary.

## E. Sarcoma: extremely rare (31 cases).

## F. Mixed mesodermal tumors

- Grossly simulate solid carcinoma.
- Microscopic: papillary pattern of an epithelial malignancy combined with a stromal malignancy or other mesodermal tissue (cartilage, rhabdomyoblast).
- Prognostic poor: life span measured in months.
- Treatment: surgery. More recently, adjunctive chemotherapy.

### Suggested Readings

1. Budowick M, Johnson TRB Jr, Genadry R, Parmley TH, Woodruff JD. The histopathology of the developing tubal ectopic pregnancy. *Fertil Steril* 34:169, 1980.
2. Denham JW, Maclennan KA. The management of primary carcinoma of the fallopian tube: Experience of 40 cases. *Cancer* 53:166, 1984.
3. Dorfman SF, Grimes DA, Cates W Jr, Binkin NJ, Kafrissen ME, O'Reilly KR. Ectopic pregnancy mortality, United States 1979 to 1980: Clinical aspects. *Obstet Gynecol* 64:386, 1984.
4. Eschenbach DA. Epidemiology and diagnosis of acute pelvic inflammatory disease. *Obstet Gynecol* 55:142s, 1980.
5. Honore LH. Salpingitis isthmica nodosa in female infertility and ectopic tubal pregnancy. *Fertil Steril* 29:164, 1978.
6. Landers DV, Sweet RL. Current trends in the diagnosis

and treatment of tuboovarian abscess. *Am J Obstet Gynecol* 151:1098, 1985.

7. Pauerstein CJ, Croxatto HB, Eddy CA, Ramzy I, Walters MD. Anatomy and pathology of tubal pregnancy. *Obstet Gynecol* 67:301, 1986.
8. Sapan IP, Solberg NS. Prolapse of the uterine tube after abdominal hysterectomy. *Obstet Gynecol* 42:26, 1973.
9. Stock RJ, Nelson KJ. Ectopic pregnancy subsequent to sterilization: Histologic evaluation and clinical implications. *Fertil Steril* 42:211, 1984.

# 8. The Ovary: Inflammations, Non-neoplastic Lesions, Abnormal Gonadal Sex Differentiation, and Premature Ovarian Failure

I. Embryology
II. Histology
III. Inflammations
IV. Non-neoplastic lesions
V. The ovary in abnormal gonadal sex differentiation
VI. The ovary in premature ovarian failure

## I. Embryology

- Ovary derives from three sources: celomic epithelium, mesenchyme, and primordial germ cells.
- The ovary is mesodermal in origin, except for the germ cells, which come from the endoderm.

**A. Celomic epithelium:** On each side, thickened area of celomic epithelium on the medial side of the mesonephros develops during the 5th week.

**B. Mesenchyme**

- Proliferation of the celomic epithelial cells and condensation of the underlying mesenchyme form the pair of gonadal ridges (genital ridges).

1. **Proliferations of cells from the celomic epithelium grow into the underlying mesenchyme.** The undifferentiated gonad at this stage consists of an outer cortex and an inner medulla. In embryos with XX chromosomes, the cortex differentiates into an ovary and the medulla regresses (10th week). Those early proliferations degenerate and disappear. Remnants form the rete ovarii.
2. **Subsequent cell proliferations** extend from the surface epithelium into the mesenchyme and incorporate the primordial germ cells (cortical cords).
3. **Cortical cords** begin to break up into isolated cell clusters and form primordial follicles at 16 weeks.

### C. Primordial germ cells

- Visible at 4 weeks among the endodermal cells of the wall of the yolk sac.
- Migrate along the dorsal mesentery of the hindgut to the gonadal ridges.
- During the 6th week, migrate into the underlying mesenchyme and become incorporated in nests of epithelial cells (primordial follicles).
- Six million germ cells present in embryos of 6–7 months, reduced to 400,000–600,000 oocytes at menarche.

## II. Histology

### A. Celomic epithelium *(surface epithelium)*

- Covers the ovary, mesodermal in origin.
- Consists of a single layer of cuboidal to low columnar epithelial cells that are separated from the underlying stroma by a distinct basement membrane.

- Can differentiate into tubal, endometrial, cervical, and transitional epitheliums.
- Is the source of most ovarian tumors.

**B. Germ cell:** large round cell with clear cytoplasm and a large vesicular nucleus, with finely dispersed chromatin and one or more nucleoli.

### C. Cortex and medulla

- *Cortex:* broad, consists of stroma made up of spindle-shaped connective tissue cells. Can become luteinized in nests and can synthesize steroids (dihydroepiandrosterone [DHEA], androstenedione, testosterone). Cortex contains follicles and their derivatives.
- *Medulla:* connective tissue matrix surrounding blood vessels, lymphatics; contains rete ovarii and hilus cells.

#### 1. Follicle

- *Primordial follicle:* central germ cell encircled by a low cuboidal layer of epithelium: membrana granulosa.
- Granulosa becomes cuboidal and stratified as the follicle grows, then shows a central cavity or antrum.
- *Mature follicles* composed of, from outside inward:
  - Theca externa.
  - Theca interna, very vascular.
  - Membrana granulosa: layers of round or polyhedral cells with dark nuclei that undergo frequent mitoses. Call-Exner bodies (clear central cavity surrounded by a layer of granulosa cells).
  - Antrum with liquor folliculi.
  - Germ cell area with
    - Cumulus oophorus or discus proligerus.

- Corona radiata.
- Zona pellucida.
- Perivitelline space.
- Ovum: vitelline membrane, germinal vesicle (nucleus), and germinal spot (nucleolus).

- *Corpus luteum of menstruation*
  - Theca interna prominent with largely ovoid or polyhedral cells (paralutein cells); produces primarily estrogens.
  - Penetration of the granulosa by vessels from the theca interna.
  - Granulosa cells become large and polyhedral with abundant, eosinophilic cytoplasm and small dark nuclei (lutein cells) forming the lutein layer. Produces primarily progesterone.
  - Layer of fibroblasts forms after post-ovulation hemorrhage into the lumen.
  - Theca interna regresses and divides the lutein zone into compartments.
  - Intraperitoneal hemorrhage may occur. (Clinical picture similar to that of ectopic pregnancy.)
  - Increased fibrosis of the lutein zone, forming a *corpus albicans* which is resorbed by the ovarian stroma.
- *Corpus luteum of pregnancy*
  - Corpus luteum becomes larger and has a cystic content with prominent lutein and paralutein cells.
  - May proliferate and become theca lutein cysts similar to those found in trophoblastic disease.
- *Atresia folliculi and corpus fibrosum.* Follicles that do not complete maturation undergo atresia: death of ovum, degeneration of granu-

losa, follicular cyst with wall formed by theca interna, cicatricial obliteration, and formation of corpus fibrosum or corpus atreticum.

2. **Ovarian changes in pregnancy**
   - Corpus luteum of pregnancy retrogresses after 2½ months.
   - Decidual cells beneath the surface of the ovary.
3. **Rete ovarii**
   - Remnant of early proliferations of surface epithelial cells in the hilum of every ovary (analogous to the rete testes).
   - Appears as narrow, slit-like tubules lined by a flat epithelium and no surrounding muscle tissue.
4. **Mesonephric tubules:** clusters of small lumina lined by cuboidal epithelium and always surrounded by a thick muscular zone.
5. **Hilus cells**
   - Polyhedral or ovoid cells arranged in mosaic fashion.
   - Present in the hilus of all ovaries.
   - Contain Reinke crystals.
   - Histologically and functionally related to the Leydig cells of the testicle.
6. **Ectopic adrenal:** Ectopic adrenal cortex tissues are found near the hilum or along ovarian vessels of 15–20% of specimens (Marchand).
7. **Ovary in menopause**
   - Absence of primordial follicles, maturing follicles, corpora lutea, and atretic follicles.
   - Stroma becomes less cellular or more hyperplastic (stromal hyperplasia).

## III. Inflammations

- Most inflammatory lesions of the ovary are on the peritoneal surfaces and are secondary to inflammations of the tube.

### A. Acute oophoritis

- Superficial, appears as a serofibrinous or fibrinous acute oophoritis.
- Can be involved with inflammations of the tube, appendix, or sigmoid.
- Treatment: antibiotics.

### B. Abscess of the ovary

- Rare.
- Occurs in patients undergoing vaginal hysterectomy or in association with pyosalpinx, occasionally with IUD.
- Microscopic: purulent exudate (polymorphonuclear leukocytes and cellular detritus) surrounded by ovarian stroma that can show locally acute inflammatory reaction.
- Deposits of cholesterol crystals.
- Pseudoxanthoma cells which can mimic lutein cells.
- Treatment: antibiotics and surgery.

### C. Chronic peri-oophoritis

- Most frequent finding in old PID.
- Gross: adherent but normal ovary.
- Microscopic: layer of connective tissue involving the ovarian surface. Metaplasia of mesothelium into cuboidal, columnar epitheliums with secretory and ciliated elements (and psammoma bodies), or into squamous epithelium (Walthard islands).
- Treatment: antibiotics and surgery.

### D. Chronic oophoritis

- Poorly defined pathologic entity.
- Microscopic: diffuse chronic inflammatory infiltration of the stroma.

## IV. Non-neoplastic lesions

### A. Epithelial inclusion cysts *(mesothelial inclusion cysts)*

- Most frequent, nonfunctional.
- Result of invaginations of the mesothelium into the ovarian stroma.
- Lined by cuboidal or low columnar cells of the surface epithelium.
- No pathologic significance if small.
- Treatment: surgery if large.

### B. Follicle cysts

- Result of atresia of follicles, often tiny but sometimes become cystic and attain 8–10 cm.
- Generally are resorbed and disappear within a few days.
- Gross: smooth surface, thin wall, contain clear watery fluid.
- Lined by granulosa cells which can become luteinized.
- Sometimes difficult to distinguish from serous cysts, and called "simple cysts."
- May persist, become functional and secrete estrogens (irregular bleeding, endometrial hyperplasia).
- Treatment: conservative observation, oral contraceptives, surgery if persistent for 6–8 weeks (cystectomy).

## C. Lutein cysts

### 1. Granulosa lutein cyst

- Most frequent: *corpus luteum cyst.*
- Cyst wall formed by granulosa lutein cells.
- Becomes *corpus albicans cyst* with hyalinization of the lutein layer.
- Can rupture and mimic ectopic pregnancy.
- Surgery if rupture (cystectomy).

### 2. Theca lutein cyst *(hyperreactio luteinalis)*

- Associated with hydatidiform mole or choriocarcinoma, rarely with normal pregnancy, or with twin pregnancy or with patients receiving gonadotropin therapy.
- Constitutes a response to the secretion of a large amount of human chorionic gonadotrophin (HCG) by the trophoblast.
- Gross: multiple, bilateral cysts that produce massive ovarian enlargement.
- Microscopic: marked luteinization of the theca interna (granulosa often not prominent).
- No treatment. Cysts will resorb after treatment of the cause.

## D. Luteoma of pregnancy

- Solid "ovarian tumor" with yellow-gray nodules composed of large, polygonal, luteinized cells.
- Can be bilateral.
- Not a true neoplasm, but an exaggerated physiologic response of the ovary to the increased endocrine stimulus of gestation.
- Associated with virilization of the mother or female fetus in 25% of cases.
- Most regress spontaneously after pregnancy.

- Treatment: solitary nodules should be excised for diagnosis; no treatment required.

## E. Polycystic ovaries *(Stein-Leventhal ovary)*

- Gross: two to five times the size of normal ovary, oyster gray; smooth firm cortex, no evidence of corpus luteum formation, small bluish cysts.
- Microscopic: thick cortical tunica, numerous cystic follicles in all stages of maturation or atresia, hyperplasia and luteinization of the theca interna that surrounds the cysts, proliferation of the medullary stroma which occasionally contains foci of lutein cells.
- Clinical: anovulation (with amenorrhea or irregular bleeding), hirsutism, obesity, elevated LH ($>$ 25 mIU/ml), low or low-normal FSH (LH/FSH ratio greater than 3), increased testosterone, androstenedione, dihydroepiandrosterone, and estrone.
- Treatment: clomiphene, medroxyprogesterone, or OCA.

## F. Hyperthecosis

- Merged imperceptibly with Stein-Leventhal (SL) syndrome but considered a different entity by some authors.
- Gross: ovaries rounded and enlarged (7 cm), thick pseudocapsule, follicle cysts. Cut section reveals pink or yellow tissue.
- Microscopic: stromal hyperplasia with clusters of lutein cells. Follicular cysts may be few or absent.
- Clinical: symptoms like those of SL patients but ovulation can't be induced with clomiphene; marked virilization.
- Treatment: as with SL patients. Wedge resection occasionally (result not permanent). TAH-BSO if patient over 35 years old and does not desire fertility.

### G. Endometrial cysts

- May be single or multiple, and with adhesions on the surface.
- Contain thick, chocolate-like fluid.
- Gross: walls of cyst dark red or brownish red.
- Microscopic: endometrial glands and stroma, hemosiderin-laden macrophages in a fibroblastic stroma and an epithelial lining.
- Treatment: surgery if large.

## V. The ovary in abnormal gonadal sex differentiation

### A. Turner's syndrome *(45XO or mosaicism)*

- Short stature, webbing of neck, low hairline, low-set ears, shield chest with widely spaced nipples, short 5th finger.
- Streak gonads (2.3 × 0.5 cm): sheets and whorls of fibrous tissue; no germ cells are present. Hilar cells and mesonephric remnants may persist.

### B. True hermaphrodism

- Most true hermaphrodites are raised as males.
- Most are chromatin positive and have a 46XX cytogenetic constitution.
- There may be testes on one side and an ovary on the other, or there may be an ovotestis.
- Gonads are usually found in abdomen; uterus is almost always present.
- Diagnosis of true hermaphrodism is made only by the anatomic demonstration of both ovarian and testicular tissues.
- Sex assignment is usually based on the external genitalia.

# VI. The ovary in premature ovarian failure

**A. True premature menopause:** ovaries without primordial or developing follicles, resemble postmenopausal ovaries.

**B. Resistant ovary syndrome:** ovaries with normal number of primary follicles but absence of developing follicles.

**C. Autoimmune oophoritis**

- Infiltration of atretic follicles, developing follicles, and corpora lutea by lymphocytes and plasma cells (theca interna layer more infiltrated than granulosa layer).
- Patients often have associated immune disorders, most frequently Addison's disease.

## Suggested Readings

1. Alper MM, Garner PR. Premature ovarian failure: Its relationship to autoimmune disease. *Obstet Gynecol* 66: 27, 1985.
2. Chang RJ, Judd HL. The ovary after menopause. *Clin Obstet Gynecol* 24:181, 1981.
3. Coney P. Polycystic ovarian disease: Current concepts of pathophysiology and therapy. *Fertil Steril* 42:667, 1984.
4. Coulam CB. Premature gonadal failure. *Fertil Steril* 38:645, 1982.
5. Garcia-Bunuel R, Berek JS, Woodruff JD. Luteomas of pregnancy. *Obstet Gynecol* 45:407, 1975.
6. Hallatt JG, Steele CH Jr, Snyder M. Ruptured corpus luteum with hemoperitoneum: A study of 173 surgical cases. *Am J Obstet Gynecol* 149:5, 1984.
7. Nagamani M, Lingold JC, Gomez LG, Garza JR. Clinical and hormonal studies in hyperthecosis of the ovaries. *Fertil Steril* 36:326, 1981.

8. Reed MJ, Beranek PA, Ghilchik MW, James VHT. Conversion of estrone to estradiol and estradiol to estrone in postmenopausal women. *Obstet Gynecol* 66:361, 1985.
9. Stein IF, Leventhal ML. Amenorrhea associated with bilateral polycystic ovaries. *Am J Obstet Gynecol* 29: 181, 1935.
10. Wetchler SJ, Dunn LJ. Ovarian abscess: Report of a case and a review of the literature. *Obstet Gynecol Surv* 40:476, 1985.

# 9. Generalities on Ovarian Neoplasms

I. Histogenetic classification of ovarian neoplasms
II. Primary ovarian neoplasms related to age
III. Symptoms of patients with ovarian cancer
IV. FIGO staging of carcinoma of ovary
V. Incidence of subclinical metastases in stages I and II ovarian carcinoma
VI. Treatment of ovarian cancer
VII. Five-year survival of epithelial ovarian cancer in relation to stage

## I. Histogenetic classification of ovarian neoplasms

### A. Neoplasms derived from celomic epithelium (65%)

1. Serous tumor (50%) (benign, borderline, malignant).
2. Mucinous tumor (25%) (benign, borderline, malignant).
3. Endometrioid tumor.
4. Clear cell (mesonephroid) tumor.
5. Brenner tumor.

6. **Undifferentiated carcinoma (15%).**
7. **Mixed mesodermal tumor.**

### B. Neoplasms derived from germ cells (20%)

1. **Dysgerminoma.**
2. **Embryonal carcinoma.**
3. **Endodermal sinus tumor.**
4. **Choriocarcinoma.**
5. **Teratomas:** mature, immature, monodermal.
6. **Gonadoblastoma.**

### C. Neoplasms derived from specialized gonadal stroma (10%)

1. **Granulosa—theca tumors.**
2. **Sertoli-Leydig tumors (arrhenoblastomas).**
3. **Gynandroblastoma.**
4. **Lipid cell tumors.**

### D. Neoplasms derived from nonspecific mesenchyme (5%)

1. **Fibroma, hemangioma, leiomyoma, lipoma.**
2. **Lymphoma.**
3. **Sarcoma.**

## II. Primary ovarian neoplasms related to age

- *Up to 20 years:* germ cell, 59%; celomic epithelium, 29%; specialized gonadal stroma, 8%; nonspecific mesenchyme, 4%.
- *From 20 to 50 years:* celomic epithelium, 71%; germ cell, 14%; nonspecific mesenchyme, 10%; specialized gonadal stroma, 5%.

- *Over 50 years:* celomic epithelium, 81%; nonspecific mesenchyme, 9%; germ cell, 6%; specialized gonadal stroma, 4%.

## III. Symptoms of patients with ovarian cancer

- Abdominal pain and swelling (50%).
- Gastrointestinal symptoms (heartburn, anorexia, nausea, bloating) (20%).
- Urinary symptoms, abnormal bleeding, weight loss.

## IV. FIGO staging of carcinoma of ovary

- *Stage I:* growth limited to the ovaries.
  - *IA:* one ovary, no ascites, no tumor on external surface; capsule intact.
  - *IB:* both ovaries, no ascites, no tumor on external surface; capsule intact.
  - *IC:* IA or IB with tumor on surface of one or both ovaries; or with capsule ruptured or with ascites containing malignant cells or with positive peritoneal washings.
- *Stage II:* growth involving one or both ovaries and with pelvic extension.
  - *IIA:* extension to uterus or tubes.
  - *IIB:* extension to other pelvic tissues.
  - *IIC:* IIA or IIB with tumor on surface of one or both ovaries, or with capsule ruptured or with ascites containing malignant cells or with positive peritoneal washings.
- *Stage III:* growth involving one or both ovaries and with intraperitoneal metastases outside the pelvis and/or positive retroperitoneal or inguinal nodes. Superficial liver metastasis.
  - *IIIA:* microscopic seeding of peritoneal cavity—nodes negative.

- *IIIB:* abdominal implants less than 2 cm—nodes negative.
- *IIIC:* abdominal implants greater than 2 cm and/or positive retroperitoneal or inguinal nodes.

- *Stage IV:* growth involving one or both ovaries and with distant metastases (pleural effusion positive for cancer, parenchymal liver metastasis).

## V. Incidence of subclinical metastases in stages I and II ovarian carcinoma (Piver et al)

| | |
|---|---|
| • Diaphragm: 15.7% | (Stage I: 11.3%)<br>(Stage II: 23.0%) |
| • Aortic nodes: 10.3% | (Stage I: 10.3%)<br>(Stage II: 10.0%) |
| • Malignant cytologic washings: 29.8% | (Stage I: 32.9%)<br>(Stage II: 12.5%) |

## VI. Treatment of ovarian cancer

**A. Surgery:** surgical staging and cytoreduction; total abdominal hysterectomy, bilateral salpingoophorectomy, omentectomy, node sampling, debulking to less than 2 cm size tumor. Second-look operation after 6–12 courses of chemotherapy. For conservative surgery in a child or a young woman, a frozen-section diagnosis of the tumor will guide management.

### B. Chemotherapy

#### 1. Celomic epithelium neoplasms

- Cisplatin, Adriamycin, cyclophosphamide (PAC) intravenously.
- Intraperitoneal chemotherapy: intraperitoneal cisplatin.

2. **Germ cell neoplasms**
   - Vincristine, actinomycin D, cyclophosphamide (VAC).
   - Vinblastine, bleomycin, cisplatin (VBP).
3. **Stromal tumors**
   - Chemotherapy not well evaluated.
   - PAC, VAC, AcFuCy (actinomycin, 5-fluorouracil, and cyclophosphamide).

**C. Radiation:** used in early stage of dysgerminoma with pelvic or aortic nodal disease.

## VII. Five-year survival of epithelial ovarian cancer in relation to stage

- Stage I, 62%.
- Stage II, 44%.
- Stage III, 13%.
- Stage IV, 4%.
- Overall 5-year survival rate, 31% (FIGO 1985).

### Suggested Readings

1. Heintz APM, Hacker NF, and Lagasse LD. Epidemiology and etiology of ovarian cancer: A review. *Obstet Gynecol* 66:127, 1985.
2. Piver MS, Barlow JJ, Lele SB. Incidence of subclinical metastasis in Stage I and II ovarian carcinoma. *Obstet Gynecol* 52:100, 1978.

# 10. Epithelial Tumors of the Ovary

I. Serous tumors
II. Mucinous tumors
III. Endometrioid tumors
IV. Clear cell tumors
V. Brenner tumors
VI. Undifferentiated carcinoma
VII. Malignant mixed mesodermal tumors

The coelomic epithelium is totipotent and can differentiate into tubal epithelium (serous tumor), endocervical or intestinal epithelium (mucinous tumor), endometrial epithelium (endometrioid and clear cell tumors), and urothelial epithelium (Brenner tumor).

## I. Serous tumors

- Constitute 20–50% of all ovarian tumors.
- Benign, 70%; borderline, 5–10%; malignant, 20–25%.
- Borderline and invasive serous tumors account for 35–40% of all ovarian cancers.

### A. Gross

1. **Serous cystadenoma:** unilocular or multilocular, thin-walled cyst with watery fluid; papillary outgrowth coarse and composed mainly of stroma. Bilateral in 7–12% of cases.

2. **Serous cystadenocarcinoma, borderline:** low malignancy potential. Difficult to distinguish from the papillary serous cystadenoma, but papillarity more lush and fine; requires differential diagnosis with microscope. Bilateral in 26% of cases. (Woodruff and Julian.)

3. **Serous cystadenocarcinoma:** cystic and papillary or entirely solid, bilateral in ⅔ of cases; friable, necrotic, hemorrhagic.

## B. Microscopic

- The cellular alterations in the papillary serous tumor usually remain constant from one area to another.
- Three types of cells
  - Flattened or round cell with abundant acidophilic cytoplasm, classic of mesothelium.
  - Ciliated.
  - Secretory, analogue to tubal epithelium.
- Psammoma bodies, often found.

1. **Benign:** one layer of cells, no malignant change of epithelium, no mitoses.

2. **Borderline:** cellular stratification, branching papillary fronds, solid cellular budding and tufting, nuclear atypicality, mitoses (never more than 1 MF/HPF—Woodruff), psammoma bodies, detachment of atypical cell clusters, absence of stromal invasion (most important). Diagnosis should be based on the ovarian tumor and not on the metastatic implants.

3. **Malignant:** invasion of stroma, formation of papillae, and presence of psammoma bodies. Proliferation of cells with disparity of cellular pattern and nuclear activity. Increased mitotic

activity (more than 1 mitosis per HPF—Woodruff).

- Histologic grading made on basis of papillary pattern (and not on epithelial lining cells): grades I, II, III (well, moderately, and poorly differentiated).

- If the tumor is predominantly stroma, it is called *serous adenofibroma*.

## C. Clinical

- Asymptomatic until lesion is large.
- Prognostic depends on the clinical stage and histologic grade of lesions.

1. **Benign serous tumors:** excellent prognosis. Occur during reproductive years and in infancy.
2. **Serous tumors of borderline malignancy:** often associated with spread beyond ovary (19–47%) in the form of peritoneal implants; late metastases (up to 30 years later) or multifocal disease.
3. **Serous carcinomas:** malignant and with extensive abdominal implantation and ascites, lymph node metastases.

## D. Treatment

- Surgery (TAH-BSO, omentectomy; second-look operation).
- No adjunctive chemotherapy in stage IA, IB tumors of borderline malignancy (Creasman).
- Chemotherapy: alkylating agents; cisplatin.

**E. Prognosis:** borderline tumors, 5-year survival, stage I, 90%; stage III, 80%. Serous carcinoma, 5-year survival, stage I, 66%; stage III, 15%.

## II. Mucinous tumors

- Constitute 15–25% of all ovarian tumors.
- Mucinous carcinomas account for 6–10% of all ovarian cancers.
- Benign, 85%; borderline, 6%; invasive, 9%.

### A. Gross

- Largest of all ovarian tumors (300 lbs recorded).
- Intraovarian, rarely papillary.
- Smooth outer surface, multilocular with thin walls, mucinous fluid thick and viscid.
- Borderline and invasive forms have papillary growth, thick and knobby (solid) areas.
- Bilaterality: 5% in benign, 10–20% in borderline and invasive forms.

### B. Microscopic

- Multiple sections necessary because there is no uniform pattern (different from pattern or serous cystadenocarcinoma).
- Characteristic tall columnar epithelium with clear cytoplasm and basally placed nuclei (endocervical epithelium).
- Goblet cells or squamous metaplasia can be seen.

1. **Benign:** single row of columnar mucinous cells.
2. **Borderline:** papillarity, epithelial stratification, budding, bridging, nuclear atypicality, absence of invasion (which is impossible or *very* difficult to determine).
    - Hart and Norris: height of the atypical epithelium, three layers or fewer.
    - Woodruff and Novak: fewer than 4 mitoses per high power field.

3. **Mucinous cystadenocarcinoma**
   - Epithelial stratification: 4 layers or more of atypical cells (Hart and Norris).
   - Mitoses: 4 or more MF/HPF (Novak and Woodruff).
   - Invasion of the stroma.
   - *Pseudomyxoma peritonei:* accumulation of gelatinous material in the peritoneal cavity due to spontaneous perforation of mucinous cysts (most are borderline).

## C. Clinical

1. **Benign:** favorable clinical course.
2. **Borderline:** can recur in the pelvis or abdomen.
3. **Mucinous carcinoma:** remains confined to ovary and pelvis for a long time, metastasizes late (5–10 years after surgery), often to lungs.

## D. Treatment

- Surgery: TAH-BSO and omentectomy in older women; unilateral salpingo-oophorectomy (USO) in young women for benign or borderline tumors.
- Chemotherapy: disappointing.
- Treatment of pseudomyxoma peritonei: no effective treatment.

## E. Prognosis

- Borderline tumors: 5-year survival, stage I, 77%; stage III, 66%. Mucinous carcinomas: 5-year survival, stage I, 66%; stage III, 20%.
- Most patients with pseudomyxoma peritonei live 5 years or more.

## III. Endometrioid tumors

- Constitute 5% of all ovarian tumors.
- Endometrioid cancers account for 15–25% of all malignant ovarian neoplasms.
- Tumors of borderline malignancy are rare, and criteria for their diagnosis have not yet been elucidated.

### A. Gross

- Endometrioid carcinomas difficult to distinguish from other ovarian cancers: solid masses with soft or fibrous consistency, or cystic with thin, velvety lining and containing chocolate-like fluid.
- Bilateral in 30% of cases.

**B. Microscopic:** adenocarcinomatous pattern like that of carcinoma of endometrium; 25–50% are adenoacanthoma. Adenosquamous tumors are rare and of poor prognosis.

### C. Clinical

- Remain confined to the ovary and pelvis; 10–15% of endometrioid carcinomas of the ovary are associated with adenocarcinoma of the endometrium.
- Rarely metastasize.

**D. Treatment:** surgery, chemotherapy, progestational agents.

### E. Prognosis

- Excellent, low-grade malignancy even in case of association with adenocarcinoma of the endometrium (two primary tumors; multifocal disease).
- Prognosis depends on the stage of the tumor.
- Five-year survival: stage I, 59%; stage III, 12%.

# IV. Clear cell tumors *(mesonephroid tumors)*

- Benign tumors are not reported.
- Borderline lesions are rare.
- Clear cell carcinomas: 5–8% of all ovarian cancers.

## A. Gross

- Large, unilateral, often unilocular.
- Smooth surface with cystic and solid components.
- Bilateral in 3% of stage I cases.

## B. Microscopic

- Two basic histologic patterns: clear cell and hobnail cell.

1. **Clear cell:** tall clear cell with basophilic nuclei; usually eccentric.
2. **Hobnail cell:** prominent bulbous nuclei protruding into the lumen; no cytoplasm, membrane collapsed about the nucleus.
   - Mitoses infrequent.
   - Can be found with other patterns, especially with endometrioid and serous carcinomas.

## C. Clinical

- Seventy-five percent of patients are over 40 years old.
- Associated with hyperpyrexia and hypercalcemia.

## D. Treatment: as for other ovarian epithelial neoplasms.

## E. Prognosis

- Five-year survival: stage I, 44%; stage III, 6%.

## V. Brenner tumors

- Constitute 2–3% of all ovarian tumors.
- Majority are benign: less than 2% are borderline or malignant.

### A. Gross

- Size: variable, primarily microscopic (⅓ of cases less than 2 cm) but occasionally of large size (8.6 kg).
- Solid like fibroma; sometimes appear as firm nodules in the wall of a mucinous cystadenoma.
- Capsule poorly defined; sectioned surface firm, hard, gray-white or white.
- Borderline tumors are predominantly cystic and multilocular.
- Bilateral in 6% of cases.

### B. Microscopic

- Characteristic nests of epithelial cells surrounded by an abundant stroma (reminiscent of Walthard rests, i.e., squamous metaplasia in a preexisting epithelial tumor—Arey).

1. **Epithelial cells:** round or cylindrical, small or bulky, very uniform, abundant pale cytoplasm, nuclei with coarse chromatin and longitudinal groove (coffee bean nucleus). In some cases, the superficial epithelium may be columnar and mucus-secreting.
2. **Stroma:** fibromatous, almost acellular. Can show hyaline changes or calcifications. Can demonstrate theca-like alterations (eosinophilic cytoplasm, large pale nucleus with well-defined nucleolus).
   - Borderline or malignant tumors: epithelium exhibits mitoses and features of atypi-

cality (carcinoma in situ and epidermoid carcinoma).

- Borderline: absence of marked cytologic atypia, confinement to ovary, similar to CIN.
- Malignant: metastasis, high-grade cytological features, destructive stromal invasion.

### C. Clinical

- No characteristic symptoms.
- Occur frequently in postmenopausal women (50% are in the 6th decade of life).

### D. Treatment

- Surgery: TAH-BSO.
- Conservative surgery in young women.

### E. Prognosis: excellent even with borderline: 95% 5-year survival. Poor with malignant variant.

## VI. Undifferentiated carcinoma

- Accounts for 15–30% of all cases of common epithelial carcinomas.
- Lacks a distinctive pattern of differentiation toward the 5 major types of epithelial carcinomas.

### A. Gross

- Differs little from poorly differentiated serous or endometrioid carcinoma.
- Solid with areas of necrosis or hemorrhage.
- Twenty-five percent of stages I and IIA are bilateral.

### B. Microscopic

- Solid masses or irregular nests or cords of epithelial cells surrounded by a stroma which may be desmoplastic.
- Tumor cells are moderate in size with all the characteristic features of malignancy.
- Giant cells, sometimes with psammoma bodies.

### C. Clinical

- Resembles serous carcinoma.
- At time of exploration 40% are at stage III.
- Lymph node spread is common.

### D. Treatment: similar to other types of epithelial tumors.

### E. Prognosis: poor; 5-year survival, stage I, 47%; stage III, 7%.

## VII. Malignant mixed mesodermal tumors

- Of 240 cases reported, 60% are heterologous.
- Median age: 58 years; 25%, less than 50 years.

### A. Gross

- Soft to firm, yellow to brown with solid areas.
- Bilateral, 10%.

### B. Microscopic

- Epithelial component: endometrioid or serous carcinoma, rarely mucinous or squamous.
- Mesenchymal component: homologous (fibrosarcoma) or heterologous (cartilage, striated muscle).

### C. Clinical: rapidly growing tumor; 50% are stage III when discovered.

**D. Treatment:** surgery, radiation, and chemotherapy (VAC).

**E. Prognosis:** poor; no more than 4 years' survival.

## Suggested Readings

1. Arey LB. The origin and form of the Brenner tumor. *Am J Obstet Gynecol* 81:743, 1961.
2. Barnhill D, Heller P, Brzozowski P, Advani H, Gallup D, Park R. Epithelial ovarian carcinoma of low malignant potential. *Obstet Gynecol* 65:53, 1985.
3. Colgan TJ, Norris HJ. Ovarian epithelial tumors of low malignant potential: A review. *Int J Gynecol Pathol* 1:367, 1983.
4. Czernobilsky B. Endometrioid neoplasia of the ovary: A reappraisal. *Int J Gynecol Pathol* 1:203, 1982.
5. Dinh TV, Slavin RE, Bhagavan BS, Hannigan EV, Tiamson EM, Yandell RB. Mixed mesodermal tumors of the ovary: A clinicopathologic study of 14 cases. *Obstet Gynecol* 72:409, 1988.
6. Hart WR, Norris HJ. Borderline and malignant mucinous tumors of the ovary: Histologic criteria and clinical behavior. *Cancer* 31:1031, 1973.
7. Hernandez E, Rosenshein NB, Bhagavan BS, Parmley TH. Tumor heterogeneity and histopathology in epithelial ovarian cancer. *Obstet Gynecol* 63:330, 1984.
8. Kurman RJ, Craig JM. Endometrioid and clear cell carcinoma of the ovary. *Cancer* 29:1653, 1972.
9. Kurman RJ, Ganjei P, Nadji M. Contributions of immunocytochemistry to the diagnosis and study of ovarian neoplasms. *Int J Gynecol Pathol* 3:3, 1984.
10. Richardson GS, Scully RE, Nikrui N, Nelson JH Jr. Common epithelial cancer of the ovary (first of two parts). *N Eng J Med* 312:415, 1985.
11. Richardson GS, Scully RE, Nikrui N, Nelson JH Jr.

Common epithelial cancer of the ovary (second of two parts). *N Eng J Med* 312:474, 1985.

12. Roth LM, Dallenbach-Hellweg G, Czernobilsky B. Ovarian Brenner tumors I: Metaplastic, proliferating and of low malignant potential. *Cancer* 56:582, 1985.
13. Silverberg SG. Brenner tumor of the ovary: A clinicopathologic study of 60 tumors in 54 women. *Cancer* 28:588, 1971.

# 11. Germ Cell Tumors of the Ovary

I. Classification and derivation of germ cell tumors
II. Dysgerminoma
III. Endodermal sinus tumor
IV. Choriocarcinoma
V. Embryonal carcinoma
VI. Polyembryoma
VII. Teratomas
VIII. Gonadoblastoma

## I. Classification and derivation of germ cell tumors (Teilum)

*Germ cell*

*Dysgerminoma* ⟵ ⟶ *Embryonal carcinoma* ⟶ *Polyembryoma?*

Extra-embryonic pathway → *Endodermal sinus tumor*, *Choriocarcinoma*

Embryonic pathway → *Teratoma*
—Mature (dermoid cyst)
—Immature
—Monodermal (struma ovarii, carcinoid)

- Constitute 20–25% of ovarian tumors.
- In patients under 21 years old, ⅔ of ovarian tumors are germ cell type (and ⅓ of these are malignant).
- Germ cell tumors may be mixed: necessary to sample all areas of the tumor exhaustively.

- Prognosis for mixed germ cell tumor depends on its most malignant element.
- *Gonadoblastoma* is included with germ cell tumors because of its histology (germ cells and gonadal stroma cells) and its propensity to give rise to germ cell tumors (dysgerminoma).

## II. Dysgerminoma

- Found in both sexes (seminoma in males) at gonadal or extragonadal sites.
- Comprises 1–2% of all ovarian neoplasms, 5–10% of all ovarian tumors occurring in the first 2 decades.

### A. Gross

- Variable size (few cm to 50 cm).
- Smooth or nodular capsule.
- Solid consistency; cut surface with grayish pink and brownish yellow areas.
- Bilateral in 10–15% (necessary to biopsy the other ovary if not normal appearing).

### B. Microscopic

- Nests of large round, ovoid, or polygonal cells that resemble primordial germ cells: clear cytoplasm and a large rounded or irregular nucleus with prominent nucleoli. Few mitoses.
- Stroma consists of fibrous trabeculae infiltrated by lymphocytes.
- Giant cells may be present.

### C. Clinical

- Age: 80–85% of patients are between 10 and 30 years old.
- Accounts for 20–30% of malignant ovarian tumors during pregnancy.

- Occasionally associated with intersex states and gonadoblastoma.
- Very sensitive to radiotherapy and chemotherapy.
- Propensity for lymphatic spread (aortic and pelvic).
- Associated with elevated levels of serum lactic dehydrogenase (LDH) and $LDH_1$.

**D. Treatment:** surgery (TAH-BSO or USO in case of small tumor stage IA) and radiation for lymphatic involvement or tumor larger than 10 cm: 75% of recurrences are eradicated with radiotherapy. Chemotherapy (VAC or VBP) in cases of peritoneal involvement and distant metastases.

**E. Prognosis:** excellent; 90–95% 5-year survival in stage I disease, 60–90% 5-year survival in all stages.

## III. Endodermal sinus tumor *(yolk sac tumor)*

- Over 350 cases reported; in one large series, yolk sac tumor constituted 22% of all germ cell lesions reported.

### A. Gross

- Solid tumor with cystic degeneration, usually unilateral.
- Soft, pultaceous, friable tissue, grayish brown.

### B. Microscopic

- Neoplastic cells: abundant and clear cytoplasm with irregular nuclei—mitoses frequent.

1. **Reticular pattern** characterized by a meshwork of communicating spaces that are lined by flat, pleomorphic, mesothelial-like cells.

2. **Endodermal sinus (Schiller-Duval body):** single central vessel lined with primitive columnar cells, lies in a space bordered by flattened, hobnail-shaped cells. May appear round (like glomerulus tuft) or elongated according to the plane of section.
3. **Hyaline granules** containing alpha-fetoprotein and $alpha_1$-antitrypsin (intracellular or extracellular, brightly eosinophilic, PAS [periodic acid Schiff] positive).

### C. Clinical

- Patients: young females, average age 16.
- Rapidly growing tumor: ⅓ have spread beyond the ovary at the time of surgery (to peritoneum, nodes, liver).
- Tumor markers: high alpha-fetoprotein (AFP) in most cases; high $alpha_1$-antitrypsin in some.

### D. Treatment: 
surgery (USO) and chemotherapy within 2 weeks of surgery; VAC (vincristine, actinomycin D, cyclophosphamide) or VBP (vinblastine, bleomycin, cisplatin)—VBP more toxic.

### E. Prognosis: 
poor before chemotherapy (95% mortality within 2 years). Improved with VAC: 90% 2-year survival, stages I and II; 50% 2-year survival, stages III and IV.

## IV. Choriocarcinoma

- Over 100 cases recorded.
- Patients under 20 years.

### A. Gross

- Most choriocarcinomas are combined with malignant germ cell tumors (immature teratomas); a few are pure.
- Solid, hemorrhagic, and friable.

### B. Microscopic

- Syncytiotrophoblast: syncytium with many dark nuclei and knots.
- Cytotrophoblast: large, rounded cells with clear cytoplasm.

### C. Clinical

- Isosexual precocity in half the cases if tumor develops before puberty.
- Irregular bleeding, enlargement of breasts.
- Tumor marker: HCG.

### D. Treatment: surgery and chemotherapy. Prognosis poor even with chemotherapy (different from that of gestational choriocarcinoma): fatal in one year with abdominal and pulmonary metastases.

## V. Embryonal carcinoma

- Reported in 1976 by Kurman and Norris (15 cases).
- Composed of embryonal cells of epithelial appearance that grow in patterns like those of embryonal carcinoma of testes.

**A. Gross:** unilateral, solid; necrotic and hemorrhagic on sectioning.

**B. Microscopic:** tumor cells large and primitive and with scattered syncytiotrophoblast and hyaline bodies, occasional glandular and papillary formations.

### C. Clinical

- Tumor markers: HCG and AFP.
- Median age of patients: 15 years (younger than patients with EST [endodermal sinus tumor]); precocious puberty, irregular uterine bleeding, amenorrhea, hirsutism.

**D. Treatment:** surgery and chemotherapy (VAC or VBP).

**E. Prognosis:** 5-year survival, 39%.

## VI. Polyembryoma

- Exceedingly rare (7 reported cases).

**A. Gross:** solid, pinkish gray mass, with areas of hemorrhage.

**B. Microscopic:** numerous embryoid bodies in varying stages of development.

**C. Prognosis:** poor survival; highly malignant neoplasm not sensitive to radiotherapy; response to chemotherapy unknown.

## VII. Teratomas

- Constitute 15% of all primary ovarian tumors.
- Recapitulate the development of the three embryonic layers.
- Ninety-five to ninety-eight percent are benign.
- Malignancy is demonstrated by the *inability of the tissue to mature,* rather than by anaplasia of individual cells.

### A. Mature teratomas

- Most are cystic (dermoid cysts); solid mature teratomas rare.
- Predominant element: ectoderm.
- Can have elements of the other 2 layers.
- Gross: cystic with smooth capsule small to 7.7 kg or 40 cm in diameter, 15–18% bilateral. Content: sebaceous material mixed with hair, cerebrospinal fluid (CSF), neural tissue, cartilage.

Rokitansky's protuberances where teeth and bone are found. Homunculus: structure representing an abortive attempt to form a fetus.

- Microscopic: ectodermal, endodermal, and mesodermal derivatives: stratified squamous epithelium with appendages; respiratory epithelium with peribronchial glands and cartilage; neural elements and endodermal epithelium (gastrointestinal epithelium, salivary gland).
- Clinical: asymptomatic. Most found in reproductive years. Rare in postmenopause. (Tumor present for years.)
- Complications: torsion (frequent, 10–12%), rupture (chemical peritonitis), infection (salmonella), autoimmune hemolytic anemia.
- Treatment: surgery (excision). Do not wedge the other ovary if it appears and feels normal.
- Prognosis: excellent.
- Malignant transformation of benign teratoma: rare (0.5%); most common malignancy—squamous cell carcinoma; salvage rate poor.

## B. Monodermal teratomas

### 1. Struma ovarii (300 cases reported)

- Thyroid tissue dominant in the tumor; constitute 2.7% of ovarian teratomas.
- Sometimes associated with carcinoid pattern, sometimes mixed with dermoid cyst.
- Gross: grayish brown, spongy, and with large cystic areas (often associated with mucinous cyst), less than 10 cm in diameter.
- Microscopic: normal thyroid tissue; only 5–10% malignancy.
- Clinical: patients in the 5th or 6th decades of life, abnormal thyroid function.
- Treatment: surgery.
- Prognosis: good if benign.

### 2. Carcinoid (200 cases reported)

- Associated with other teratomatous components in 95% of cases.
- Has been mistaken histologically for granulosa cell tumor or arrhenoblastoma because of the cord-like or tubular arrangement of the cells.
- Gross: small, tan nodule that protrudes in the lumen of a dermoid cyst.
- Microscopic
  - *Insular carcinoid:* islands of neoplastic cells lie in a fibroma-like stroma. Nuclei are round and uniform in size. Small round acini are present in the islands with intraluminal eosinophilic secretion.
  - *Trabecular carcinoid:* long, wavy parallel ribbons of cells, 1–2 cells thick, in a fibrous stroma.
  - *Strumal carcinoid:* admixture of thyroid tissue and carcinoid.
- Clinical:
  - *Insular carcinoid:* ⅓ have carcinoid syndrome. Treat as an ovarian cancer with a limited potential for spread. Monitor 5-HIAA (hydroxyindoleacetic acid).
  - *Trabecular carcinoid:* treat as an ovarian cancer with low malignant potential.
  - *Strumal carcinoid:* treat as an ovarian tumor of very low malignant potential.
- Prognosis: good; 5% recur in insular and trabecular carcinoids, 2% recur in strumal carcinoids (Robboy and Scully). If bilateral, probably metastatic.

## C. Immature teratomas

- Rare; 0.2% of all ovarian tumors, less than 1% of ovarian teratomas.

- Criteria for malignancy: immature elements.
- Gross: solid, lobulated masses with many small cysts. Solid tissue includes cartilage, bone; soft gray or cream-colored tissue represents immature neural tissue; never bilateral.
- Microscopic: Tissues of all three germ layers are found, immature or mature. Predominant tissue: neural (neuroepithelium in the form of rosettes and tubules, glial tissue with atypical cells, areas resembling neuroblastoma).
- Grading I to III according to the degree of differentiation and the quantity of immature tissue (Scully-Norris)
  - *Grade 0:* wholly mature tissue.
  - *Grade 1:* abundant mature tissue but some immaturity (glial tissue, primitive mesenchyme); neuroepithelium absent or 1 LPF (×40) per slide.
  - *Grade 2:* greater immaturity; neuroepithelium not exceeding 3 LPF per slide.
  - *Grade 3:* severe immaturity; neuroepithelium 4 or more LPF per slide.
- Clinical: Prognosis related to stage and grade.
- Occurs most commonly in the first 2 decades of life; unknown after menopause.
- Tumor spread in the abdomen in ⅓ of cases, occasionally in the form of mature glial implants (better prognosis).
- Distant metastases rare.
- Treatment: surgery (unilateral salpingo-oophorectomy with sampling of peritoneal implants) and chemotherapy VAC (vincristine, actinomycin D, cyclophosphamide) or MAC (methotrexate, actinomycin D, chlorambucil). Chemotherapy can cause "chemotherapeutic retroconversion" of immature teratoma into mature elements.
- Survival: at 5 years, 64% for all stages.

## VIII. Gonadoblastoma

- Mixed tumor with germ cell and gonadal stroma tumor elements.
- Almost all patients have underlying abnormalities in gonadal development and sex chromosomes (46XY; 45X/46XY).
- Age range: 6–38 years.
- Gross: largest lesion 8 cm, either soft and fleshy or firm and cartilaginous; contain granules of calcification; ¼ are microscopic tumors; ⅓ are bilateral.
- Microscopic
  - Germ cells.
  - Sex cord derivatives that resemble immature Sertoli and granulosa cells (very small, round or oval, pale nuclei devoid of mitotic activity).
  - Germ cells and immature granulosa or Sertoli cells grow in nests which contain hyaline bodies and calcifications.
  - Leydig (or lutein) cells between the nests, and in the stroma in ⅔ of cases.
- Invasive dysgerminoma develops from a gonadoblastoma in half the cases.
- Clinical
  - Hormonal effect generally androgenic.
  - Treatment: bilateral gonadectomy if Y chromosome.
  - Prognosis: excellent, in case of pure gonadoblastoma; reserved, in case of dysgerminoma or other germ cell tumor associated with gonadoblastoma.

### Suggested Readings

1. Genadry R, Parmley TH, Woodruff JD. Secondary malignancies in benign cystic teratomas. *Gynecol Oncol* 8:246, 1979.
2. Gershenson DM, DelJunco G, Herson J, Rutledge FN.

Endodermal sinus of the ovary, the M.D. Anderson experience. *Obstet Gynecol* 61:194, 1983.

3. Gershenson DM, Copeland LJ, Kavanagh JJ, Cangri A, DelJunco G, Saul PB, Stringer CA, Freedman RS, Edwards CL, Wharton JT. Treatment of malignant nondysgerminomatous germ cell tumors of the ovary with vincristine, dactinomycin and cyclophosphamide. *Cancer* 56:2756, 1985.
4. Gordon A, Lipton D, Woodruff JD. Dysgerminoma: A review of 158 cases from the Emil Novak Ovarian Tumor Registry. *Obstet Gynecol* 58:497, 1981.
5. Kurman RJ, Norris HJ. Embryonal carcinoma of the ovary. *Cancer* 38:2420, 1976.
6. Kurman RJ, Norris HJ. Endodermal sinus tumor of the ovary. *Cancer* 38:2404, 1976.
7. Norris HJ, Zirkin HJ, Benson WL. Immature (malignant) teratoma of the ovary: A clinical and pathologic study of 58 cases. *Cancer* 37:2359, 1976.
8. Scully RE. Ovarian tumors of germ cell origin. *Prog Gynecol* 5:1340, 1971.
9. Scully RE. Gonadoblastoma: A review of 74 cases. *Cancer* 23:1340, 1970.
10. Takashina T, Kanda Y, Hayakawa O, Kudo R, Ito E, Sagae S. Yolk sac tumors of the ovary in the human yolk sac. *Am J Obstet Gynecol* 156:223, 1987.
11. Talerman A, Haije WG, Baggerman L. Serum alphafetoprotein (AFP) in diagnosis and management of endodermal sinus (yolk sac) tumor and mixed germ cell tumors of the ovary. *Cancer* 41:272, 1978.
12. Taylor MH, Depetrillo AD, Turner AR. Vinblastine, bleomycin and cisplatin in malignant germ cell tumors of the ovary. *Cancer* 56:1341, 1985.

# 12. Gonadal Stromal Tumors of the Ovary


I. Classification
II. Granulosa cell tumors
III. Theca cell tumors (thecomas)
IV. Sertoli-Leydig cell tumors
V. Gynandroblastoma
VI. Lipid cell tumors


## I. Classification

- Granulosa cell tumors.
- Thecomas (theca cell tumors).
- Sertoli-Leydig cell tumors (arrhenoblastomas, androblastomas).
- Gynandroblastoma (rare).
- Lipid cell tumors:
  - Hilus cell tumor.
  - Adrenal-like cell tumor.
- Have been classified as sex-cord stromal tumors or mesenchymomas.
- Account for 6–10% of all ovarian tumors.
- No adequate correlation of tumor morphology and endocrine effect.

## II. Granulosa cell tumors

- Fewer than 2% of ovarian tumors.

### A. Gross

- Size: several mm to 69 kg.
- Often unilateral, smooth outer surface, sometimes lobulated.
- Cut surface solid gray or yellow; cystic cavities contain fluid or clotted blood.

### B. Microscopic

- Extreme variability of pattern.
- Morphologic resemblance to granulosa cells.
- Normally associated with theca cells.
- Histologic types

1. **Folliculoid:** microfolliculoid or macrofolliculoid pattern resembles primitive follicles. Call-Exner bodies: small rounded cavities that contain an eosinophilic material.
2. **Diffuse or parenchymatous:** sea of closely packed oval, round, or angular nuclei that can exhibit prominent grooves.
3. **Pseudo-adenomatous:** arrangement resembling adenoma.
4. **Insular:** island of well-differentiated granulosa cells.
5. **Cylindroid** ***(trabecular):*** columns of granulosa cells.
6. **Watered silk:** mosaic of sinuous rows of granulosa cells.
7. **Luteinized:** large, round cells with abundant eosinophilic cytoplasm and prominent cell borders, resemble granulosa lutein cells.

8. **Juvenile granulosa cell tumors**
   - Large, immature-appearing granulosa and theca cells.
   - Abundant cytoplasm rich in lipids (luteinization).
   - Nuclei dark, rarely grooved, often with mitotic figures.
   - Call-Exner bodies rare.

## C. Clinical

- Estrogen-producing tumors.

1. **Prepubertal patients:** ¾ of granulosa cell tumors are associated with sexual pseudo-precocity (first sign: enlargement of breasts).
2. **Reproductive age:** irregular uterine bleeding due to cystic hyperplasia of the endometrium (unopposed estrogen).
3. **Postmenopausal patients:** uterine bleeding.
   - Association of granulosa theca cell tumors with endometrial carcinoma: 5–10%.
   - Capsule can rupture with intraperitoneal hemorrhage.
   - Low-grade-malignancy tumor: recurrences are late (5–20 years) and localized to abdomen or pelvis.
   - Juvenile granulosa cell tumor: observed in first 2 decades; low-grade malignancy, good prognosis. Can occur in infants with abnormal karyotypes and ambiguous genitalia.

## D. Treatment

- Unilateral salpingo-oophorectomy for stage IA in young patients.
- TAH-BSO in older women.
- Recurrences can appear very late (5–20 years);

treated with radiation, surgery, or chemotherapy (VAC or doxorubicin).

- Five-year survival: 89% if tumor is confined to ovary; 58% if extraovarian extension.

## III. Theca cell tumors (thecomas)

- Fewer than 1% of all ovarian tumors.

**A. Gross:** firm and fibrous, solid, yellowish hue, often unilateral; cyst formation is rare.

**B. Microscopic:** bands of broad, plump spindle-shaped cells with round nuclei and pale vacuolate cytoplasm, separated by connective tissue, fat-stain positive (different from fibroma). Luteinized thecoma contains scattered islands of large, round, polyhedral cells that resemble theca lutein cells.

**C. Clinical**

- Rare before puberty, frequent before menopause and after.
- Three times more often associated than granulosa cell tumors with an abnormal endometrium.
- Benign, except in rare cases of malignant thecoma.

**D. Treatment:** unilateral oophorectomy if patient is young, TAH-BSO if menopausal. Prognosis is good.

## IV. Sertoli-Leydig cell tumors *(arrhenoblastomas, androblastomas)*

- Account for 0.2% of all ovarian tumors.

**A. Gross:** moderate size or small, almost always unilateral; surface smooth, cut surface grayish yellow and firm and with frequent cystic degeneration.

**B. Microscopic:** complex.

1. **Well-differentiated form:** tubules with lumen lined by well-differentiated columnar cells. Cells contain oval, dark nuclei and moderate amount of eosinophilic cytoplasm. Leydig cells between tubules (testicular adenoma of Pick).
2. **Intermediate form:** masses, nests, or cords of Sertoli cells together with Leydig cells (Reinke crystalloids).
3. **Undifferentiated form:** sarcoma-like picture with cord-like arrangement of cells, imperfect-tubule formation.
4. **With heterologous elements:** endodermal (mucinous cysts) or mesodermal (skeletal muscle, cartilage, etc.).

**C. Clinical**

- Typically produce androgens and virilize 70–80% of patients.
- Virilization occurs more with intermediate and undifferentiated forms.
- Clinical signs of defeminization, then masculinization: oligomenorrhea, atrophy of breasts, acne, hirsutism, clitoromegaly, deepening of voice.
- Plasma androgens: high levels of testosterone and androstenedione, but normal or slightly elevated DHEA.
- A small proportion of Sertoli-Leydig cell tumors are associated with estrogenic manifestations.
- Low-grade malignancy. Poorly differentiated tumors have poor prognosis. Recurrences appear early. Stages higher than I have a poor prognosis (mortality 100% in Young and Scully's series).

### D. Treatment

- Unilateral salpingo-oophorectomy in stage IA tumors.
- Five-year survival, 70–90%.

## V. Gynandroblastoma

- Rare tumor that contains granulosa or theca cells together with Sertoli or Leydig cells.
- Masculinizing effect predominates.
- Low-grade malignancy.

## VI. Lipid cell tumors

### A. Hilus cell tumor *(Leydig cell tumor)*

- *Gross:* always small (less than 5 cm), unilateral, yellow or brown.
- *Microscopic:* Leydig cells with Reinke crystalloids in cytoplasm.
- *Clinical:* virilization, but endometrium often shows an estrogenic effect (10% associated with adenocarcinoma of endometrium). Occurs generally in perimenopause.
- Benign tumor.

### B. Adrenal-like tumor

- Rare and benign.
- Can be from gonadal stromal origin, or from aberrant adrenal tissue.
- Microscopic: large polygonal clear cells like adrenal cortical cells.
- Symptoms of virilization if tumor large.

## Suggested Readings

1. Dinh TV, Fougerousse CL, Nagamani M. Hormonal studies on adrenal-like tumor of the ovary: Considerations on its histogenesis. *Am J Clin Pathol* 86:388, 1986.
2. Dunnihoo DR, Grieme DL, Woolf RB. Hilar cell tumors of the ovary: Report of 2 new cases and a review of the world literature. *Obstet Gynecol* 27:703, 1966.
3. Evans AT, Gaffey TA, Malkasian GD Jr, Annegers JF. Clinicopathologic review of 118 granulosa and 82 theca cell tumors. *Obstet Gynecol* 55:231, 1980.
4. Ireland K, Woodruff JD. Masculinizing ovarian tumors. *Obstet Gynecol Survey* 31:83, 1976.
5. Jacobs AJ, Deppe G, Cohen CJ. Combination chemotherapy of ovarian granulosa cell tumor with cis-platinum and doxorubicin. *Gynecol Oncol* 14:294, 1982.
6. Lack EE, Perez-Atayde AR, Murthy ASK, Goldstein DP, Crigler JF, Vawter GF. Granulosa theca cell tumors in premenarchal girls: A clinical and pathologic study of ten cases. *Cancer* 48:1846, 1981.
7. Stenwig JT, Hazekamp JT, Beecham JB. Granulosa cell tumors of the ovary: A clinicopathological study of 118 cases with long term follow-up. *Gynecol Oncol* 7:136, 1979.
8. Taylor HB, Norris HJ. Lipid cell tumors of the ovary. *Cancer* 20:1953, 1967.
9. Young RH, Scully RE. Ovarian Sertoli-Leydig cell tumors: A clinicopathological analysis of 207 cases. *Am J Surg Pathol* 9:543, 1985.
10. Young RH, Scully RE. Ovarian sex cord-stromal tumors: Recent advances and current status. *Clin in Obstet Gynecol* 11:93, 1984.

# 13. Miscellaneous Tumors of the Ovary

- I. Fibroma
- II. Ovarian sarcomas
- III. Lymphoma
- IV. Small cell carcinoma
- V. Metastatic lesions

## I. Fibroma *(fibrothecoma)*

- Occurs in the 5th and 6th decades of life.

### A. Gross

- Small size when seen as polypoid growths on ovarian surface, but can be enormous and weigh 50 lbs. Tumor should be larger than 3 cm to be categorized as fibroma.
- Dense and solid, bilaterality 4–8%.
- Cut surface whitish and homogeneous. Areas of cystic degeneration are seen in large tumors, which often develop pedicles (torsion).

### B. Microscopic

- Fusiform cells with abundant cytoplasm and pale nucleus (functional cells) or spindle-shaped cells with small, round, dark nuclei that resemble fibrocytes.
- Hyalinization frequent, calcification possible.

### C. Clinical

- Pelvic tumor.
- Meig's syndrome: ovarian fibroma, hydrothorax, and ascites.
- Gorlin's syndrome (basal nevus syndrome): hereditary disorder characterized by keratocysts of the jaw, basal cell carcinomas, and ovarian fibromas (often bilateral and calcified).

### D. Treatment

- Benign tumor: unilateral salpingo-oophorectomy or TAH-BSO.

## II. Ovarian sarcomas

- Rare; incidence compared to carcinoma is 1 to 40.
- More common in the adult than in the young child.

**A. Teratoid sarcoma:** in young patients under 25 years; admixture of bizarre tissues representing histologic variations from all germ layers; can arise from a benign teratoma (leiomyosarcoma, fibrosarcoma).

**B. Stromal cell sarcoma or fibroleiomyosarcoma:** arise from fibromas or fibrothecomas (greater than 4 MF/10 HPF: very poor prognosis—Woodruff-Scully).

**C. Mixed mesodermal tumor:** See Chapter 10. Prognosis poor.

## III. Lymphoma

- Primary extranodal lymphomas of the ovary are rare.
- Nearly always secondary to a primary gastrointestinal lesion.

- All varieties of lymphomas have been described (Hodgkin's disease, Burkitt's tumor, non-Hodgkin lymphomas, poorly differentiated types). Burkitt's lymphoma frequently affects the ovary.
- Ovarian involvement by leukemia: 30–50% cases.
- Treatment is that for lymphoma in general: surgery with postoperative radiation or chemotherapy.
- Five-year survival rate, 10%.
- Tumor often bilateral—ovarian tissue replaced by malignant lymphoma cells.

## IV. Small cell carcinoma

- Eighty cases published by Young and Scully.
- Average age: 22 years (10–42 years).
- Symptoms: abdominal pain and swelling.
- Gross: tumor unilateral and with white or tan masses.
- Microscopic: sheets of small epithelial cells with scanty cytoplasm and small nuclei with small nucleoli; numerous mitoses.
- Hypercalcemia in ⅔ of cases.
- Very poor prognosis.
- Treatment: TAH-BSO. Chemotherapy or radiation unsuccessful.
- Origin of tumor still unknown.

## V. Metastatic lesions

### A. Primary genital tumors

#### 1. Adenocarcinoma of the endometrium

- Most commonly associated with an ovarian malignancy (4.8%).
- Five-year survival 50%. High survival rate demonstrates that adenocarcinomas of ovary and endometrium are in truth two primary tumors.

2. **Cervical carcinoma:** rarely metastasizes to the ovary (1%).
3. **Tubal carcinoma**
   - May involve ovary (13%).
- Gross: metastatic ovarian lesion small.
- Microscopic: resemble the original carcinoma (endometrium, cervix, or tube).

## B. Primary extragenital tumors

1. **Breast primary tumor**
   - Twenty-five percent of ovarian metastases occur in association with recurrent breast cancer.
   - Both ovaries are involved in 60–80%.
   - Gross: tumors solid, mobile, bosselated.
   - Microscopic: cortical portion most often involved.
   - Variety of patterns
     - Like that of primary breast lesion.
     - Small columns of metastatic cancer in ovarian stroma: Indian file.
     - Sometimes signet cells as in Krukenberg tumor.
   - Clinical: most patients die within 1 year.
2. **Gastrointestinal primary tumor**
   - Gross: solid, bilateral, lobulated, and free; sometimes tremendous size (2,000 g); can be cystic in case of metastasis from large intestine. Section friable, mushy yellow-red or gray tissue.
   - Microscopic: variety of microscopic patterns sometimes accurately replicating a mucinous ovarian primary tumor (small or large glands with mucin-containing goblet cells). Stroma can be edematous or desmoplastic.

- Clinical: 20% of GI tumors metastasize to ovaries.
- Most patients die within 3 years.

### C. Krukenberg tumor of the ovary

- Gross: solid, bilateral, reniform; external surface white, smooth, with capsule; cut surface variegated: firm, spongy, cystic, hemorrhagic. Ovarian tumor size often overshadows the gastrointestinal lesion.
- Microscopic
  - Stroma is cellular in one area, edematous or myxomatous in others.
  - Epithelial elements occur in clusters of acini with mucoid change: large number of signet ring cells (nucleus flattened against cell wall).
- Clinical
  - Abdominal pain, swelling, abnormal uterine bleeding.
  - Most Krukenberg tumors are secondary to lesions of the stomach (30%), large intestine, and breast; rarely, when they are primary, they have a better prognosis (5–13 year survival).
  - Nearly all patients die within 1 year.

## Suggested Readings


1. Azoury RS, Woodruff JD. Primary ovarian sarcomas: Report of 43 cases from the Emil Novak Ovarian Tumor Registry. *Obstet Gynecol* 37:920, 1971.
2. Dickersin GR, Kline IW, Scully RE. Small cell carcinoma of the ovary with hypercalcemia: A report of eleven cases. *Cancer* 49:188, 1982.
3. Dockerty MB, Masson JC. Ovarian fibromas: A clinical and pathologic study of two hundred and eighty-three cases. *Am J Obstet Gynecol* 47:741, 1944.

4. Holtz F, Hart WR. Krukenberg tumor of the ovary: A clinicopathologic analysis of 27 cases. *Cancer* 50:2438, 1982.
5. Joshi VV. Primary Krukenberg tumor of ovary: Review of literature and case report. *Cancer* 22:1199, 1968.
6. Meigs JV. Fibroma of the ovary with ascites and hydrothorax—Meigs' syndrome. *Am J Obstet Gynecol* 67:962, 1954.
7. Woodruff JD, Murthy YS, Bhaskar TN, Bordbar F, Tseng SS. Metastatic ovarian tumors. *Am J Obstet Gynecol* 107:202, 1970.
8. Young RH, Carey RW, Robboy SJ. Breast carcinoma masquerading as primary ovarian neoplasm. *Cancer* 48:210, 1981.

# 14. Diseases of the Mesosalpinx and Uterine Ligaments

I. Mesosalpinx
II. Round ligament
III. Broad ligament

## I. Mesosalpinx

- Contains the paraovarium, remnant of the wolffian body, which consists of a main mesonephric duct and a group of 12–16 tubules extending towards the hilum of the ovary.
- Cysts of various sizes can arise from the mesonephric duct and tubules. Histology: lumen lined by a single layer of cuboidal epithelium and surrounded by a layer of muscle tissue.
- Most gross cystic lesions represent dilatation of accessory lumina of the tube: lumen are lined by typical tubal epithelium (ciliated and nonciliated cells).
- Paraovarian cysts: situated between tube and ovary; lined by cuboidal or columnar epithelium in a single layer; arise rarely from mesonephric elements (3 out of 116 cysts—Genadry et al); most represent mesothelial inclusions or tubal accessory lumina; malignant degeneration rare (4 out of 116 cases). The hydatid of Morgagni is the most common paramesonephric cyst.

## II. Round ligament

- Benign tumors: fibromyoma, adenomyoma, cysts of the canal of Nuck (dilatations of the peritoneal investment of the round ligament).
- Malignant tumors: sarcoma, carcinoma; rare.

## III. Broad ligament

- Leiomyoma, lipoma.
- Tumors that arise from mesonephric rests (ovarian tumor of probable wolffian origin: 12 cases—2 developed metastases—Young and Scully).
- Hilar cell and adrenal rest tumors (see Chapter 12).

### Suggested Readings

1. Gardner GH, Greene RR, Peckham B. Tumors of the broad ligament. *Am J Obstet Gynecol* 73:536, 1957.
2. Genadry R, Parmley T, Woodruff JD. The origin and clinical behavior of the paraovarian tumor. *Am J Obstet Gynecol* 129:873, 1977.
3. Samaha M, Woodruff JD. Paratubal cysts: Frequency, histogenesis and associated clinical features. *Obstet Gynecol* 65:691, 1985.
4. Young RH, Scully RE. Ovarian tumors of probable wolffian origin: A report of 11 cases. *Am J Surg Pathol* 7: 125, 1983.

# 15. The Placenta

I. Embryology
II. Normal placenta
III. Abnormalities
IV. The placenta in disease
V. Inflammations
VI. Benign tumor: chorioangioma
VII. Malignancies: gestational trophoblastic disease
VIII. Secondary neoplasms

## I. Embryology

- Placenta has two components: (1) maternal portion formed by the endometrium; (2) fetal portion developed from the chorion.
- *Maternal portion:* decidua basalis (endometrium underlying the conceptus; the other two regions are the decidua parietalis and the decidua capsularis, which will fuse together at 22 weeks).
- *Fetal portion:* chorionic plate and villi that arise from it.
- Villi cover entire chorionic sac up to 8 weeks of pregnancy.
  - Villi associated with decidua capsularis degenerate and produce the chorion laeve (smooth chorion).
  - Villi associated with decidua basalis proliferate, branch, and form the chorion frondosum (villous chorion). The latter in direct contact with the decidua basalis continues to develop and forms the placenta.

## II. Normal placenta

- Discoid organ 15–20 cm in diameter, 2–3 cm in thickness.
- Weight approximately 450 g; ratio of weight of placenta to that of fetus at term—1:6 to 1:7.
- Implantation site: Nitabuch's stria, which is a fibrinoid deposit at the interface of the trophoblast (villi) and maternal tissue (decidua).
- Syncytial endometritis and myometritis: individual trophoblastic cells invade the myometrium and endometrium, can simulate choriocarcinoma (intermediate trophoblast).
- Involution of placental site: hyalinized small arteries.
- Trophoblast consists of
  - Cytotrophoblast: composed of Langhans cells, which are cuboidal cells with clear cytoplasm, round or oval light-staining nuclei; progenitor of syncytiotrophoblast and intermediate trophoblast. Contains no human placental lactogen and human chorionic gonadotropin.
  - Syncytiotrophoblast: composed of large cells with darker-staining cytoplasm and multiple nuclei; produces HCG, placental lactogen, estrogen, and progesterone.
  - Intermediate trophoblast: composed of mononucleated or multinucleated cells with basophilic cytoplasm which infiltrates wall of spiral arteries or forms plugs in lumen; produces more human placental lactogen than HCG.
- Villous trophoblast: composed mostly of cytotrophoblast and syncytiotrophoblast with small amount of intermediate trophoblast.
- Extravillous trophoblast (decidua, myometrium, and spiral arteries of placental site): composed mostly of intermediate trophoblast with a small amount of cytotrophoblast and syncytiotrophoblast.

## A. Maternal surface

- Fifteen to twenty cotyledons divided by septa, in contact with decidua basalis.

**1. Villi**

a. First trimester: villi are large (170 microns) and have a loose stroma, thin-walled vessels (with nucleated red blood cells), and Hofbauer cells (placental macrophages); villi are covered by a prominent cytotrophoblastic inner layer and a syncytiotrophoblastic outer layer.

b. Second trimester: villi smaller and more numerous, stroma denser, and fetal capillaries more prominent (70 microns).

c. Third trimester: inner cytotrophoblast less conspicuous; syncytial knots; villi smaller (40 microns); no Hofbauer cell; prominent dilated capillaries.

**2. Hydropic degeneration of villi**

- Occurs in fetal death.
- Villi show reduced vascularity, are swollen and filled with fluid; only a few villi are involved (molar change is diffuse).
- Trophoblast reduced or absent (by contrast, hydatidiform mole has trophoblastic proliferation).

**3. Placental infarcts**

- Common; occur late in pregnancy.
- Located usually at the margin of the placenta.
- Site varies from a few mm to several cm; color varies from deep red (in recent infarct) to yellow white (in old infarct).
- Caused by interference with maternal circulation.

- Microscopic: intervillous deposition of fibrin, loss of nuclear staining of villi (ghost villi).
- Clinical: occurs in normal placentas but more often associated with pathologic pregnancies (toxemia, hypertension, diabetes mellitus, systemic lupus erythematosus [SLE]).

### B. Fetal surface membranes

#### 1. Amnion

- Innermost of the membranes, cuboidal epithelium.
- Thin, transparent, glistening structure.

#### 2. Chorion

- Thick, vascular, and more opaque than amnion.
- Contains ghost villi and scant decidua at its outermost margin.

#### 3. Subchorionic fibrin deposition

- Small nodules or large collections of gray-white fibrin-like substance beneath the chorionic plate.
- No clinical significance.

### C. Cord

- Mean length 60 cm.
- Contains 2 arteries and 1 vein surrounded by Wharton's jelly.
- Outer surface covered by amnion.

## III. Abnormalities

### A. Abnormalities of architecture

#### 1. Circumvallate or circummarginate placenta

- Characterized by a thick, round, white, opaque ring around the periphery of the placenta.

- Due to lateral extension of villous tissue beyond the reflection of the "chorion laeve" off the fetal surface: chorionic plate is smaller than basal plate.
- Associated with an increased incidence of antepartum hemorrhage, intrauterine growth retardation (IUGR), premature labor.
- Common cause of mid-trimester abortions (Hertig).

2. **Succenturiate lobe *(or accessory lobes)***
   - Can be single or multiple.
   - Connected to the principal portion of the placenta by vessels and membranes.
   - Clinical
     - Vasa praevia, can rupture and be fatal to the fetus.
     - Retained in utero after delivery of the main placenta.
     - Succenturiate lobe may be implanted low (placenta praevia) with subsequent premature separation.

3. **Placenta membranacea**
   - Most of the membranes are covered by placental tissue which is thin.
   - Complications: placenta praevia.

## B. Twin placentas

- Frequency of twins: 1 in 90 births; ⅓ are monozygotic. Frequency of monozygotic twinning is relatively constant worldwide (3.5 in 1,000 pregnancies).
- Gross examination of twin placentas should include a careful scrutiny of the combined membranes.
- *Monozygotic twins (identical twins):* placenta can be monochorionic and monoamnionic, mono-

chorionic and diamnionic, or dichorionic and diamnionic.

- *Dizygotic twins (fraternal twins):* dichorionic and diamnionic placenta only.

1. **Dichorionic diamnionic twin placenta**
   - Frequency: 80% of twin gestations.
   - Fetuses can be monozygotic or dizygotic.
   - If fetuses are of different sexes, they are dizygotic (fraternal) twins; if fetuses are of same sex, zygosity can be established only by genotypic studies.
   - Combined membranes opaque.
   - Microscopic: 2 chorions interposed between 2 amnions.
   - Vascular anastomoses are absent.
2. **Monochorionic diamnionic twin placenta**
   - Frequency: 20% of twin gestations.
   - Monozygotic fertilization.
   - Fetuses of same sex (identical) optimal candidates for organ transplantation.
   - Combined membranes are transparent.
   - Microscopic: no chorion between 2 amnions.
   - Vascular anastomoses can exist between the 2 fetal circulations (twin transfusion syndrome, acardiac monster, fetus papyraceus).
3. **Monochorionic monoamnionic twin placenta**
   - Extremely rare type of monozygotic fertilization.
   - Fetuses identical.
   - Frequent vascular anastomoses and intertwining of cords (perinatal loss 40%).
   - No combined membranes separating the twins.

## C. Abnormalities of membranes and cord

### 1. Amnion nodosum

- Gross: 2–3 cm gray-white, slightly elevated nodules on the amnionic surface, near the insertion of the cord, easily removed.
- Due to surface deposits of fetal squamous cells (vernix).
- Microscopic: amorphous material, fibrillary structures and poorly defined cells above the amnion.
- Clinical: Potter's syndrome—amnion nodosum, oligohydramnios, and renal aplasia.
- Should be distinguished from squamous metaplasia (granules *not* easily removed, no clinical significance).

### 2. Absence of one umbilical artery

- Frequency: 1% of all umbilical cords, 6% of the cords of at least one twin.
- Associated with congenital anomalies (esophageal atresia and imperforate anus) in 20–40% of cases.

### 3. Velamentous insertion of cord

- Cord implanted on the membranes, away from the margins of the placenta.
- Vessels can cross the internal os and become vasa praevia (hemorrhage during delivery).

### 4. Battledore placenta

- Marginal insertion of the cord.
- No clinical significance.

## D. Abnormalities of implantation and separation

### 1. Placenta praevia

- Implantation of placenta across the internal os: complete placenta praevia.

- Often there is a premature separation at time of dilatation of the internal os or thinning of the lower segment.
- Microscopic: decidua destroyed by hemorrhage and infiltration of leukocytes.

2. **Ectopic pregnancies**
   - Tubal pregnancies: 80% in ampulla, 13% in isthmus.
   - Microscopic: villi and trophoblast in lumen or walls of tube.
   - Ovarian pregnancy: rare.
   - Arias-Stella phenomenon in endometrium in 60% of cases; but the endometrium can assume any morphology of the normal phases of the endometrium.

3. **Placenta accreta**
   - Placenta attached directly to uterine muscle without intervening decidua.
   - Placenta increta and percreta: placenta penetrates to myometrium (increta) or to the serosa (percreta).
   - Microscopic: decidua basalis absent at the implantation site, Nitabuch's layer thin or absent, uterine muscle hyalinized.
   - Clinical: antepartum bleeding (association with placenta praevia), uterine rupture, failure of placental separation during third stage of labor.

4. **Abruptio placentae**
   - Premature separation of the placenta after the 20th week.
   - Abruption can be central or marginal, partial or total.
   - Gross examination is of crucial importance in the diagnosis of abruptio placentae: zone of

hemorrhage that extends into the placental tissue and replaces it.
- Microscopy adds little to the diagnosis.
- Marginal sinus rupture: separation of the placenta at its margin, classified as one form of partial abruptio.
- Clinical: association with toxemia, hypertension, trauma. Signs: pain, shock, uterine rigidity, fetal distress or death, hypofibrinogenemia, acute renal failure.

## IV. The placenta in disease

### A. Toxemia of pregnancy

- No pathognomonic histologic lesions.
- Frequent lesions are vascular: extensive placental infarction and retroplacental hematoma.
- Gross: small placenta often stained with meconium.
- Microscopic: acute and chronic infarcts (aggregation of villi with obliteration of the intervillous space); acute atherosis in maternal arterioles of the decidua (fibrinoid necrosis of vessel walls, accumulation of lipid-containing macrophages, perivascular mononuclear infiltrate); high number of syncytial knots in non-infarcted zones (Tenney-Parker's sign or "checkerboard" appearance).

### B. Erythroblastosis fetalis

- Enlarged and edematous placenta; fetus/placenta ratio 3:1 or less.
- Gross: heavy placenta with large, pale, yellow-gray, friable cotyledons.
- Microscopic: villi enlarged.
  - Trophoblast immature relative to the stage of gestation: thick syncytium with persistence of cytotrophoblast.

- Villous stroma edematous and hyperplastic; numerous Hofbauer cells; vessels decreased in number, dilated with nucleated erythrocytes (normally, nucleated erythrocytes not seen in villi after midgestation).

## C. Tuberculosis

- Rare.
- Gross: small gray firm areas on fetal surface sometimes showing caseation (tubercles).
- Microscopic: proliferation of endothelial cells, multinucleated giant cells, tubercle bacilli.

## D. Syphilis

- Rare.
- Gross: large and boggy placenta with pale, large, greasy, and friable cotyledons.
- Microscopic: villi large and club-shaped; stroma with extensive fibrosis; diminution of fetal vessels; endarteritis; focal or generalized villous immaturity. Such changes are however not pathognomonic of syphilis and can be degenerative after fetal death.
- Spirochetes can be found in such placentas and can penetrate the placental barrier at any time during pregnancy.

## E. Diabetes mellitus

- Gross: placenta may appear bulky and edematous. Likelihood of single umbilical artery is increased (3–5%).
- Microscopic: no specific features; villous immaturity, villous edema, cytotrophoblastic cell proliferation.

## V. Inflammations

### A. Amnionitis and chorionitis

- Frequent finding (10% of all deliveries).
- Ascending infection can reach membranes directly, or infection can come through the placenta via maternal circulation.
- Most common organisms: Escherichia coli and Staphylococcus.
- Microscopic: inflammatory cells in chorion and beneath amnion.

### B. Placentitis

- Villous placental tissue can be involved secondarily after membranes, or infectious agents can reach the placenta through the maternal blood.
- Microscopic: infiltration of villi by inflammatory cells (villitis).
- Listeria monocytogenes bacilli: microabcesses within villi, membranes, and fetal organs.
- Toxoplasmosis: lymphocytic infiltration of villi; organisms found in section of membranes.
- Cytomegalovirus: intranuclear inclusion with necrosis of villous stroma.

## VI. Benign tumor: chorioangioma

- Most common benign tumor of the placenta.
- Round, firm, reddish purple, encapsulated, size can vary (5 cm or smaller).
- Microscopic: well-differentiated capillary pattern of benign endothelium and fibrous tissue with chorionic stromal cells; capillaries contain fetal blood.
- Clinical: rare cause of placental inefficiency, associated with hydramnios, fetal anomalies, premature birth.

# VII. Malignancies: gestational trophoblastic disease *(GTD)*

- *Classification of gestational trophoblastic disease*
  1. **Hydatidiform mole**
     a. Complete (classic).
     b. Partial.
  2. **Invasive mole.**
  3. **Choriocarcinoma.**
  4. **Placental site trophoblastic tumor.**
- *Clinical stages of gestational trophoblastic disease*
  - *Stage I:* GTD confined to the uterine corpus.
  - *Stage II:* GTD extends to adnexae and genital structures.
  - *Stage III:* GTD extends to lungs with or without genital tract involvement.
  - *Stage IV:* other metastatic sites.

## A. Hydatidiform mole *(complete or partial)*

- Frequency: 1/2500 pregnancies in U.S., 1/125 in Taiwan.
- Gross: mass of vesicles variable in size (around 1 cm in diameter); fragments of normal placenta may be seen in partial mole.
- Microscopic
  - Hydropic swelling of villi.
  - Complete absence or scantiness of fetal blood vessels.
  - Proliferation of trophoblast that involves cytotrophoblast, intermediate trophoblast, and syncytiotrophoblast.
- Clinical: vaginal bleeding, preeclampsia prior to 24 weeks' gestation, hyperthyroidism, uterus larger than date, theca lutein cysts, high HCG, snowstorm pattern on ultrasound. Eighty percent of patients have an uncomplicated course; 20%

will progress to invasive mole, rarely to choriocarcinoma.

- Treatment: suction curettage; hysterectomy if patient is multiparous.

- *Differences between complete hydatidiform mole and partial hydatidiform mole*
  - Complete mole: androgenetic origin; karyotypes XX (96%) and XY (4%); hydropic villi with no embryo, malignant transformation 18%.
  - Partial mole: maternal contribution; karyotype: aneuploidy (triploidy most frequent); hydropic villi with normal villi; embryo cord or fetal membranes; scalloping of villi, trophoblastic inclusions; malignant transformation 2.1% (Kaju and Ohama).
  - Followup: serial HCG titers (complete moles and partial moles).
  - Partial moles account for 25% of all molar pregnancies.

## B. Invasive mole *(chorioadenoma destruens)*

- Virtually impossible to diagnose from curettings alone; diagnosis often made from hysterectomy specimens.
- Microscopic: hydropic villi invading the myometrium; excessive trophoblastic proliferation.
- Clinical: persistence of bleeding and high HCG after evacuation of mole; tumor localizes to uterus, rarely metastasizes to lungs, vagina, or vulva; severe vaginal or intraperitoneal hemorrhage.
- Treatment: chemotherapy with or without hysterectomy.
- Prognosis good; mortality 5–10%.

## C. Choriocarcinoma

- Malignant tumor due to uncontrolled growth of the trophoblast.

- Fifty percent preceded by mole, 30% by abortions, 20% by normal pregnancies.
- Gross: soft, hemorrhagic tumor.
- Microscopic: absence of villi and proliferation of intermediate, cytotrophoblast, and syncytiotrophoblast; hemorrhage, necrosis.
- Clinical: bleeding, high HCG, metastases to lungs, brain, kidneys, liver, small intestines, spleen, and vagina.
- Treatment: chemotherapy (actinomycin D, methotrexate, chlorambucil).
- Prognosis in nonmetastatic trophoblastic disease: nearly 100% cure rate; metastatic trophoblastic disease, 80% cure rate.
- Poor prognostic parameters: long duration of disease (interval since last pregnancy longer than 4 months), high pretreatment HCG titers (more than 40,000 mIU/ml), brain or liver metastasis, significant prior chemotherapy, gestational trophoblastic neoplasia after term pregnancy.

## D. Placental site trophoblastic tumor

- Described by Kurman, Norris, and Scully in 1976.
- Rarest form of gestational trophoblastic disease.
- Can be confused with choriocarcinoma.
- Gross: polypoid mass intracavitary or, most often, intramural.
- Microscopic: intermediate trophoblast consisting of sheets of large polyhedral mononucleate cells with pleomorphic nuclei and amphophilic cytoplasm. No dimorphic cell population of cytotrophoblast and syncytiotrophoblast; no hemorrhage or necrosis; strongly positive for human placental lactogen. Poor prognosis if mitotic count exceeds 4 mitotic figures per 10 high power fields (Scully).

- Clinical: amenorrhea, or vaginal hemorrhage, uterus enlarged to 8–16 week size, positive pregnancy test in ⅓ of cases, D&C results often in uterine perforation (5 out of 12 cases), low HCG.
- Responds poorly to chemotherapy.
- Prognosis good with hysterectomy (50 cases, 6 deaths).
- Considered as an extreme degree of placental site reaction (syncytial myometritis).

## VIII. Secondary neoplasms

### A. Placental metastases from maternal neoplasms

- Metastases to the placenta are blood-borne and occur only in patients with widely disseminated disease.
- In decreasing order of frequency: malignant melanoma, and carcinomata of the breast and bronchus.
- Placenta in malignant melanoma: tumor deposits visible as black or brown nodules of varying size within the placental substance. Microscopic: sheets of malignant melanoma cells in intervillous space.

### B. Placental metastases from fetal neoplasms

- Rare, from neuroblastoma.
- Bulky, pale, heavy placenta (1,000 g).
- Microscopic: plugging of fetal villous vessels by nests of neuroblastomatous cells.

**Suggested Readings**

1. Benirschke K. Examination of the placenta. *Obstet Gynecol* 18:309, 1961.

2. Berkowitz RS, Goldstein DP, Bernstein MR. Natural history of partial molar pregnancy. *Obstet Gynecol* 66:677, 1985.
3. Breen JL, Neubecker R, Gregori CA, Franklin JE. Placenta accreta, increta, percreta. *Obstet Gynecol* 49:43, 1977.
4. Czernobilsky B, Barash A, Lancet M. Partial moles: A clinicopathologic study of 25 cases. *Obstet Gynecol* 59:75, 1982.
5. Dao AH, Rogers CW, Wong SW. Chorioangioma of the placenta: Report of 2 cases with ultrasound study in one. *Obstet Gynecol* 57:46S, 1981.
6. Fox H. Morphological changes in the human placenta following fetal death. *J Obstet Gynaec Brit Cwlth* 75:839, 1968.
7. Kurman RJ, Scully RE, Norris HJ. Trophoblastic pseudotumor of the uterus: An exaggerated form of "syncitial endometritis" simulating a malignant tumor. *Cancer* 38:1214, 1976.
8. Lathrop JC, Lauchlan S, Ramakrishna N, Ambler M. Clinical characteristics of placental site trophoblastic tumor. *Gynecol Oncol* 31:32, 1988.
9. Lurain JR, Brewer JI, Torok EE, Halpern B. Gestational trophoblastic disease: Treatment results at the Brewer Trophoblastic Disease Center. *Obstet Gynecol* 60:354, 1982.
10. Kurman RJ, Main CS, Chen HC. Intermediate trophoblast: A distinctive form of trophoblast with specific morphological, biochemical and functional features. *Placenta* 5:349, 1984.
11. Naeye RL, Peters EC. Causes and consequences of premature rupture of fetal membranes. *Lancet* 1:192, 1980.
12. Scully RE, Young RH. Trophoblastic pseudotumor: A reappraisal. *Am J Surg Pathol* 5:75, 1981.
13. Surwit EA, Alberts DS, Christian CD, Graham VE. Poor prognosis gestational trophoblastic disease: An update. *Obstet Gynecol* 64:21, 1984.

14. Szulman AE, Surti U. The syndromes of hydatidiform mole I: Cytogenetic and morphologic correlations. *Am J Obstet Gynecol* 131:665, 1978.
15. Szulman AE, Surti U. The syndromes of hydatidiform mole II: Morphologic evolution of the complete and partial mole. *Am J Obstet Gynecol* 132:20, 1978.
16. Zhang J, Kraus FT, Aquino TI. Chorioamnionitis: A comparative histologic bacteriologic and clinical study. *Int J Gynecol Pathol* 4:1, 1985.

# Index


Abscess, ovary, 97
Acrochordon, 11
Actinomycosis
  cervix, 43
  endometrium, 59
  tube, 85
Adenoacanthoma, ovary, 114
Adenocarcinoma
  cervix, 50
    clear cell, 52
    endocervical, 51
    endometrioid, 51
    in situ, 50
    microinvasive, 51
    minimal deviation, 51
  clear cell
    cervix, 52
    vagina, 33
  endometrium, 67–69
    adenoacanthoma, 67
    ciliated, 67
    clear cell, 68
    endometrioid, 67
    with endometrioid carcinoma, ovary, 69
    papillary, 67
    papillary serous, 68
    secretory, 67
  vagina, 36
Adenoepidermoid carcinoma, cervix, 52
Adenoid basal carcinoma, cervix, 53
Adenoid cystic carcinoma, cervix, 53
Adenoma, cervix, 45
Adenomatoid tumor
  fallopian tube, 86
  uterus, 74
Adenomyosis, 71
Adenosarcoma, uterus, 78
Adenosis
  cervix, 45
  vagina, 33
Adenosquamous carcinoma
  cervix, 52
  endometrium, 68
  ovary, 114
Adrenal, ectopic, 96
Adrenal-like tumor, ovary, 137
Alpha feto protein
  in embryonal carcinoma ovary, 125
  in endodermal sinus tumor, 124
Alpha 1 antitrypsime, 124
Amnionitis, 157
Amnion nodosum, 153
Androblastoma, ovary, 135
Androstenedione in Sertoli Leydig tumor, 136
Arias Stella reaction
  in adenosis vagina, 33
  in cervix, 41
  in ectopic pregnancy, 154
  in endometrium, 59
  in fallopian tube, 82
  in metaplastic tumor, tube, 87
Arrhenoblastoma, ovary, 135
Atresia folliculi, 95
Auspitz's sign, 3
Autoimmune oophoritis, 102

Bartholin's
  duct cyst, 10
  glands, 1
Behcet's disease, 4
Bowenoid papulosis, 16
Bowen's disease, 15
Breast, accessory, 13
Brenner tumor, ovary, 116
Breslow's depth of invasion in melanoma, 23

Calymmatobacterium granulomatis, 7
Cambium layer, 37
Canal of Nuck cyst, 10
Carcinoid, ovary, 128
Carcinoma in situ
  vagina, 35
  vulva, 15

Caruncle, urethra, 28
Celomic epithelium, 92, 93
Cervical intraepithelial neoplasia, 45
Cervicitis
  chronic, 42
  tuberculous, 42
Cervix, metastatic carcinoma, 54
Chancre, vulva, 5
Chancroid vulva, 6
Chlamydia
  cervix, 43
  trachomatis, 7
Chorioadenoma destruens, 159
Chorioangioma, 157
Choriocarcinoma, 160
  cervix, 54
  fallopian tube, 90
  ovary, 124
  vagina, 38
Chorion
  frondosum, 147
  laeve, 147
Chorionitis, 157
Clark's levels in melanoma, 23
Clear cell carcinoma
  endometrium, 68
  ovary, 115
Condyloma
  acuminata
    cervix, 45
    urethra, 28
    vagina, 34
    vulva, 9
  giant, of Buschke and Lowenstein, 21
  lata, vulva, 6
Corpora cavernosa, 2
Corpus fibrosum, 95
Corpus luteum
  menstruation, 95
  pregnancy, 95
Corpus spongiosum, 2
Cortex, ovary, 94
Crohn's disease, vulva, 4
Cytotrophoblast
  in choriocarcinoma ovary, 125
  in placenta, 148

Decidua
  basalis, 147
  capsularis, 147
  parietalis, 147
Dermatitis, vulva
  chronic, 3
  contact, 3
Diabetes
  mellitus, 5
  placenta of, 156
Dihydrotestosterone in lichen sclerosus, 14
Donovan bodies, 7
Donovanosis, 7
Duct
  paraurethral, 27
  Skene's, 27
Dysgerminoma, 122
Dystrophy
  hyperplastic, 14
  mixed, 14

Ectopic pregnancy, 154
Embryonal carcinoma, ovary, 125
Endocervix
  histology, 40
  pregnancy, 41
Endodermal sinus tumor
  ovary, 123
  vagina, 37
Endolymphatic stromal myosis, 74
Endometrial cysts, 101
Endometrioid tumor, ovary, 114
Endometrioma, vulva, 13
Endometriosis
  cervix, 44
  fallopian tube, 87
  ovary, 101
  vagina, 33
Endometritis
  acute, 60
  chronic, 61
  postmenopausal, 61
  tuberculous, 61
Endometrium, carcinoma
  with clomiphene, 60
  dating, 57
  grading, 66
  with oral contraceptive, 60
  with progestin, 60
  proliferative phase, 58
  secretory phase, 58
  staging, 65
Epidermal inclusion cyst, vagina, 11

Epidermoid carcinoma
  cervix, 48
  endometrium, 68
  vagina, 35
Epithelial inclusion cyst, ovary, 98
Erythroblastosis fetalis, 155
Erythroplasia of queyrat, vulva, 15
Exocervix
  histology, 40
  pregnancy, 41

Fallopian tube, prolapsed, 34, 86
Fibroma
  ovary, 139
  vulva, 11
Fibrosarcoma, vagina, 37
FIGO Staging
  cervical cancer, 48
  endometrial cancer, 65
  ovarian cancer, 106
  vaginal cancer, 35
  vulvar cancer, 17
Foam cells, endometrium, 64
Folds, urogenital, 1
Follicle
  cyst, 98
  mature, 94
  primordial, 94
Fox Fordyce disease, vulva, 9

Gartner's duct cyst, 32
Germ cell tumor of ovary, classification, 121
Gestational trophoblastic disease
  classification, 158
  clinical stages, 158
Glands
  apocrine, 2
  Bartholin, 1
    in adenocystic carcinoma, 22
  holocrine, 2
  major vestibular, 2
  merocrine or eccrine, 2
  minor vestibular, 2
  suburethral, 27
Glassy cell carcinoma, cervix, 52
Gonadal stromal tumor ovary, classification, 133
Gonadoblastoma, 130
  in dysgerminoma, 123
Gorlin's syndrome, 140
Granular cell myoblastoma, vulva, 12
Granuloma inguinale, vulva, 7
Granulosa cell tumor ovary, 133
  histologic types, 133
Granulosa lutein cyst, 99
Gumma, vulva, 6
Gynandroblastoma, ovary, 137

Hemangioma, vulva, 11
Hemophilus ducreyi, 6
Hermaphrodism, 101
Herpes, 8
Herpes simplex
  cervix, 43
  vagina, 31
  vulva, 8
Hidradenitis suppurativa, vulva, 9
Hidradenoma, vulva, 12
Hilus cell
  ovary, 96
  tumor, 137
Hobnail cell, ovary, 115
Human chorionic gonadotropin
  in choriocarcinoma ovary, 125
  in embryonal carcinoma, 125
Human papilloma virus
  bowenoid papulosis, 16
  condyloma acuminata, 9
Hyaline bodies
  in embryonal carcinoma, 125
  in endodermal sinus tumor, 124
Hydatid of Morgagni, 145
Hydatiform mole
  complete, 158
  invasive, 159
  partial, 159
Hydropic degeneration villi, 149
Hydrosalpinx, 84
Hypercalcemia
  in clear cell tumor ovary, 115
  in small cell carcinoma ovary, 141
Hyperplasia, endometrium
  adenomatous, 63
  atypical, 63
  complex, 64
  cystic, 62
  simple, 64
Hyperpyrexia in clear cell tumor ovary, 115
Hyperthecosis, ovary, 100

Immature teratoma
  grading, 129
  ovary, 128
Intertrigo, vulva, 3
Intrauterine device, endometrium, 59

Juvenile granulosa cell, 134

Koilocytotic atypia, 42
Krukenberg tumor ovary, 143

Lactic dehydrogenase, serum, 123
Leiomyoblastoma, uterus, 73
Leiomyoma, 72
  bizarre, 73
  cellular, 73
  cervix, 44
  epithelioid, 73
  fallopian tube, 87
  myometrium, 72
  secondary changes, 73
  vagina, 34
Leiomyomatosis
  intravenous, 72
  peritonealis disseminata, 73
Leiomyosarcoma
  cervix, 53
  uterus, 76
  vagina, 37
Leydig cell
  in gynandroblastoma, 137
  in hilus cell tumor, 137
  in Sertoli Leydig tumor, 136
Lichen
  planus, vulva, 4
  sclerosus, vulva, 14
Lipid cell tumor, ovary, 137
Lipofibroma, vulva, 11
Liposarcoma, uterus, 79
Luteal phase defect, 59
Luteoma, ovary, 99
Lymphangiosarcoma, uterus, 79
Lymphogranuloma venereum, vulva, 7
Lymphoma, ovary, 140

Malignant mixed mesodermal tumor
  cervix, 53
  fallopian tube, 90
  ovary, 118
  uterus, 77
Marsupialization, 10
Maturation index, 31
Mucinous cyst, vagina, 33
Medulla, ovary, 94
Meig's syndrome, 140
Melanoma
  vagina, 36
  vulva, 23
Mesonephric
  ducts, 30
    adenoma, 45
    in cervix, 41
  tubules, ovary, 96
Metaplasia
  cervix, 41
  endometrium, 64
  eosinophilic, 64
  mucinous, 64
  squamous, 64
  tubal, 64
Metaplastic tumor, fallopian tube, 87
Metastatic carcinoma
  adenocarcinoma endometrium, 141
  breast carcinoma, 142
  cervical carcinoma, 142
  gastrointestinal carcinoma, 142
  in ovary, 141
  tubal carcinoma, 142
Microglandular hyperplasia, 45
  in adenosis, 33
Microinvasive carcinoma
  cervix, 46
  vulva, 18
Molluscum contagiosum, vulva, 8
Monilia
  vagina, 31
  vulva, 5
Mucinous tumor ovary
  benign, 112
  borderline, 112
  malignant, 113
Mucus cyst, vagina, 10
Müllerian ducts
  cervix, 40
  endometrium, 57
  fallopian tube, 81
  vagina, 30
Munro absess, vulva, 4

Nabothian cyst, 44
Nevi, vulva, 12
Nitabuch's stria, 148
  in placenta accreta, 154

Oophoritis
  acute, 97

auto-immune, 102
chronic, 98
Ovarian
carcinoma
staging, 106
symptoms, 106
treatment, 107
neoplasms
age, 105
classification, 104
tumor of probable Wolffian origin, 146
Ovary
menopause, 96
premature menopause, 102
resistant ovary, 102

Paget's disease, vulva, 16
Papilloma
fallopian tube, 87
urethra, 28
Paraovarian cyst, 145
Perioophoritis, chronic, 97
Placenta
abruptio, 154
accreta, 154
battledore, 153
circumvallate, 150
dichorionic diamnionic, 152
membranacea, 151
monochorionic diamnionic, 152
monochorionic monoamnionic, 152
praevia, 153
succenturiate, 151
in twin, 151
Placental
infarct, 149
metastases
from fetal neoplasms, 161
from maternal neoplasms, 161
site trophoblastic tumor, 160
Placentitis, 157
cytomegalovirus infection, 157
listeriosis, 157
toxoplasmosis, 157
Polycystic ovaries, 100
Polyembryoma, ovary, 126
Polyp
endocervical, 44
endometrial, 61
vaginal, 34
Potter's syndrome, 153
Pox virus, 8
Pregnancy, ovarian changes, 96
Premature ovarian failure, 102
menopause, 102
Primordial germ cells, 93, 94
Psammoma bodies
in serous tumor ovary, 110
in undifferentiated carcinoma ovary, 118
Psoriasis, vulva, 3
Pyosalpinx, 83

Reinke crystalloid, 137
Resistant ovary syndrome, 102
Rete ovarii, 96
Rhabdomyosarcoma uterus, 79

Salpingitis
acute, 83
chronic, 83
granulomatous, 85
isthmica nodosa, 84
lipogranulomatous, 85
subacute, 83
tuberculous, 85
Sarcoma
botryoides
cervix, 53
vagina, 37
cervix, 55
fallopian tube, 90
ovary, 140
uterus, 75
heterologous, 75
homologous, 75
mixed mesodermal, 75
mixed pure, 75
pure, 75
stromal, 77
Schiller Duval bodies
ovary, 124
vagina, 37
Schwannoma, vulva, 12
Seborrheic keratosis, vulva, 13
Serous cystadenoma
cystadenocarcinoma, 110
ovary, 109
ovary, borderline, 110
Sertoli Leydig cell tumor, ovary, 135
Small cell carcinoma, ovary, 141
Squamous
cell carcinoma in situ, vulva, 15
hyperplasia, vulva, 14

metaplasia
in adenosis, 33
in cervix, 41
Stein-Leventhal ovary, 100
Stromal nodule, uterus, 74
Stromatosis, uterus, 74
Struma ovarii, ovary, 127
Subchorionic fibrin deposition, 150
Swellings, labioscrotal, 1
Syncitio trophoblast
in choriocarcinoma ovary, 125
in embryonal carcinoma, 125
Syphilis
placenta, 156
vagina, 32
vulva, 5
Syringoma, vulva, 13

Tampon ulcer, 32
Teratoma ovary
immature, 128
mature, 126
monodermal, 127
Testosterone
cream, 14
free, 14
in Sertoli Leydig tumor, 136
Theca
cell tumor, ovary, 135
lutein cyst, ovary, 99
Tinea cruris, vulva, 3
Toxemia, pregnancy, 155
Treponema pallidum, 5
Trophoblast
cytotrophoblast, 148
extravillous, 148
intermediate, 148
syncitiohophoblast, 148
villous, 148
Tubal
carcinoma, 87
pregnancy, 85
Tubercle, genital, 1
Tuberculosis
placenta, 156
vulva, 5
Tubo-ovarian abscess, 60
Turner's syndrome, 101
Twins
dizygotic, 152
monozygotic, 151

Umbilical artery, 150, 156
Undifferentiated carcinoma, ovary, 117
Uremia, 5
Urethra
adenocarcinoma, 28
choriocarcinoma, 28
lymphoma, 28
melanoma, 28
sarcoma, 28
squamous carcinoma, 28
transitional cell carcinoma, 28
Urethral meatus, eversion, 27
Urethritis cystica, 27
Urogenital sinus, 26, 30

Vaginal inclusion cysts, 33
Vaginitis, 31
children, 31
emphysematosa, 31
postmenopausal, 32
Velamentous insertion of cord, 153
Verrucous carcinoma, vulva, 21
Vestibular adenitis, 10
Vestibule, 1
Vulva
adenocarcinoma, 22
adenocystic carcinoma, 22
basal cell carcinoma, 22
choriocarcinoma, 24
hypernephroma, 24
invasive squamous cell carcinoma, 20
malignant lymphoma, 24
melanoma, 23
microinvasive carcinoma, 17
poorly differentiated, 21
sarcomas, 23
fibrosarcoma, 24
leiomyosarcoma, 24
neurofibrosarcoma, 24
rhabdomyosarcoma, 24
superficially invasive squamous cell carcinoma, 20
verrucous carcinoma, 21
well-differentiated keratinizing, 20
Vulvar intraepithelial neoplasia, 15

Wharton's jelly, 150
Word catheter, 10

Yolk sac tumor, ovary, 123